Research in the Nursing Care of Elderly People

WILEY SERIES ON DEVELOPMENTS IN NURSING RESEARCH

Series Editor

Jenifer Wilson-Barnett
Professor of Nursing Studies and Head of Department, King's College, University of London

Volume 1
Recovery from Illness
JENIFER WILSON-BARNETT and MORVA FORDHAM, *Lecturer in Nursing Studies, King's College, University of London*

Volume 2
Nursing Research: Ten Studies in Patient Care
Edited by
JENIFER WILSON-BARNETT

Volume 3
Psychiatric Nursing Research
Edited by
JULIA BROOKING
Lecturer in Nursing Studies, King's College, University of London

Volume 4
Research in Preventive Community Nursing Care
Edited by
ALISON WHILE
Lecturer in Nursing Studies, King's College, University of London

Volume 6
Nursing Issues in Terminal Care
Edited by
JENIFER WILSON-BARNETT and JENNIFER RAIMAN, *Education Advisor, Cancer Relief Macmillan Fund*

WILEY SERIES ON
DEVELOPMENTS IN NURSING RESEARCH
VOLUME 5

Research in the Nursing Care of Elderly People

edited by

PAULINE FIELDING
Director of Nursing Services
Whipps Cross Hospital
Leytonstone
London, UK

A Wiley Medical Publication

JOHN WILEY & SONS
Chichester · New York · Brisbane · Toronto · Singapore

Library of Congress Cataloging-in-Publication Data:

Research in the nursing care of elderly people.
    (Wiley series on developments in nursing research;
v. 5) (A Wiley medical publication)
    Includes index.
    1. Geriatric nursing. I. Fielding, Pauline.
II. Series. III. Series: A Wiley medical publication.
[DNLM: 1. Geriatric Nursing. W1 W153LF v.5 /
WY 152 R432]
RC954.R47   1987   610.73′65   87–10459

ISBN 0 471 91576 9

British Library Cataloguing in Publication Data:

Research in the nursing care of elderly
    people.—(Wiley series on developments
    in nursing research).—(A Wiley medical
    publication).
    1. Geriatric nursing.—Research
    I. Fielding, Pauline
    610.73′65′072   RC954

ISBN 0 471 91576 9

Phototypeset by Input Typesetting Ltd., London SW19 8DR
Printed and bound in Great Britain by Biddles, Guildford

List of Contributors

DENIS ANTHONY, 130 Borneo Street, Walsall, West Midlands.

K. ELIZABETH BARNES, Dept. Geriatric Medicine, St Pancras Hospital, St Pancras Way, London NW1 0PE

JOHN and SENGA BOND, Health Care Research Unit, 21 Claremont Place, Newcastle upon Tyne, NE2 4AA

JANE DAWSON, School of Nursing, Queen Alexandra Hospital, Cosham, Portsmouth PO6 3LY

MANDY FADER, Geriatric Research Unit, St Pancras Hospital, St Pancras Way, London NW1 0PE

PAULINE FIELDING, Director of Nursing Services, Whipps Cross Hospital, Leytonstone, London E11 1NR

JANE FOSTER, 66 Asylum Road, Peckham, London SE15 2LW

ANDRÉE LE MAY, 16 College Road, Isleworth, Middlesex, TW7 5DH

JENIFER NEWMAN, Dept. Geriatric Medicine, The Middlesex Hospital, Mortimer Street, London W1

SALLY REDFERN, Department of Nursing Studies, Kings College (KQC), 552 Kings Road, London SW10 0UA

ANGELA SYMONS, 36 Broomhill Way, Albrook, Eastleigh, Hampshire

Contents

Series Preface

Developments in Nursing Research

Nursing science is derived from an integration of knowledge in other disciplines and from original nursing research studies. As more relevant research is completed key areas are developing, benefiting from different approaches in various patient care settings. The purpose of this series is to publish literature reviews and original material in such areas to promote nursing progress and knowledge.

Jenifer Wilson-Barnett

Introduction

It is tempting to suggest that geriatric nursing has come of age. Certainly the last twenty years have seen a growing and strengthening of that body of knowledge relating to nursing old people and as it has developed, so we have been able to witness its complexity and appreciate the extent to which much of it is still unknown.

There has been an appreciation too of the fact that old people are cared for not only in hospitals by nurses, but in community homes by care staff, in their own homes by district nurses or in their families' homes by relatives.

The nursing of old people demands a high level of knowledge about a wide range of topics which all have a bearing on this exciting speciality. These can be considered in three broad areas. Firstly, the physical aspects of care require an understanding of the physical ageing process, the effect of multiple pathology and the body's response to stress of varying kinds. Secondly, contingent upon the ageing process, psychological aspects of care demand an appreciation of mental processes which accompanying ageing. These are often extremely susceptible to the type of care given and yet frequently receive little attention in their own right. Thirdly, care is always given in some kind of social framework which may reflect wider social policies or political expediencies which in turn will indicate those values and attitudes attached to old people in society.

Research into the nursing care of old people is as diverse as the specialty itself. It spans a wide range of methodologies and shares many of the problems associated with gerontological research. For example, the use of age as a variable will disguise many unknown and unexplained processes in old peoples' development and adaptation to circumstances and events. A reliance on tools of measurement which have been standardized on younger populations will lead to problems of validity, interpretation and generalization and ethical problems may surround the need for informed consent, particularly with demented or mentally impaired old people.

All these issues are addressed in this volume. The contributors represent a wide span of interest — some of them are involved day to day in the care of old people, some are teachers, some are researchers. Not all aspects of care could be covered in one volume but this book is an attempt to look critically at some aspects of care and in so doing may help to create the positive outcome of improved quality of life that old people are due.

Research in the Nursing Care of Elderly People
Edited by P. Fielding
© 1987 John Wiley & Sons Ltd

CHAPTER 1

The Accurate Measurement of Pressure Sores

DENIS ANTHONY

Introduction

In a system of assessing the progress of a sore, one requires some idea of change of size, as well as details such as whether the sore is infected, necrotic, oedematous, etc. Waterlow (1985) describes a system using a record sheet, where one data item is the size of a sore. How should one produce the measurement, however?

It is apparently a simple task to determine the size of a pressure sore. The lesions are certainly very much larger than the scale in which scientists and engineers routinely work. It is the purpose of this chapter to explore methods used previously to achieve this end, and to look at a new method utilizing a microcomputer.

The accuracy of sore measurement is not generally considered. It is thought that current methods produce acceptable results. It is common in clinical practice to trace decubitus ulcers using a felt pen and transparent medium. If one can see the difference in successive tracings when placed one over another, it might be thought that this will show the technique valid. Unfortunately this is not the case. For if the sore does not change size, and the tracing method is inaccurate, one will possibly get the same result, i.e. tracings which look different from one week to the next.

What is needed is more work on the validity of various techniques used to record changes. This is a general point, not restricted to pressure sores. The whole of this chapter has relevance beyond ulcer measurement, and certain diversions will deliberately be taken. If some of the more mathematical aspects do not interest you, or cause difficulty, they may be omitted with little loss. The appendix on the digitizer described towards the end of the chapter, and the computer program may easily be ignored unless one requires to use the method, and to adapt it to other computers or digitizers.

Methods of Measurement

Diameters

One Diameter

The easiest way to calculate size is to measure the diameter of a sore. But what is a diameter? One definition is 'a straight line passing through the centre of a circle or other figure, terminated at both ends by the circumference' (*Chambers Everyday Dictionary*, 1975). This gives a single measurement, but there are a choice of candidates to use as a diameter, except in perfectly circular sores. One way to overcome this problem of definition of a diameter, is to choose the longest diameter. A ruler or tape-measure may be adequate for this task. Peter Lowthian has used cut circles of measured diameter, which are placed over the sore. Thus the sore is recorded as greater or less than the area of the circle. A set of such stencils could be used to bracket the size of a sore, assuming it is roughly circular.

David (1984) used a single diameter, as did Barton and Barton (1973), David gave no indication of the accuracy of this technique. Barton and Barton stated that the measurements were done to an accuracy of one-tenth of an inch. This is probably the smallest division of the ruler used. Barnes and Malone-Lee (1985) measured pressure sores with a ruler to a stated 0.1 cm. This was the smallest scale on the ruler.

The specific disadvantage of using only one diameter is that a long thin sore of the same area as a rounder sore, will appear larger on this scale. Alternatively a sore that heals on its short axis will not be noted to change.

Two Diameters

To surmount the above problem some workers measure two diameters. The longest and shortest diameters are commonly employed. Rhodes *et al.* (1979) measured longest and shortest diameters with a transparent ruler. In both cases the ruler went through the mid-point of the lesion.

They stated that as far as was possible the same nurse took the measurements. This is important, as shall be shown later.

In addition they used the diameters to calculate area by the formula:

$$\text{Area} = \text{PI} * (\text{long axis}/2) * (\text{short axis}/2) \qquad (1)$$

(*Note*: The symbol '*' is used instead of 'X' as the multiplication symbol throughout this chapter, and in the computer program.)

It might appear that taking an average diameter, dividing by two to obtain a radius, squaring, and multiplying by the number 'PI' would give the same area.

$$\text{Area} = \text{PI} * \text{square of (average diameter}/2) \qquad (2)$$

This is of course the familiar formula for deriving the area of a circle:

$$\text{Area of circle} = \text{PI} * \text{square of radius} \qquad (3)$$

For the special case of a circle both formulae (1) and (2) yield identical results (both correct). As the sore increases its ratio of longest to shortest diameter the formulae diverge. Formula (2) becomes increasingly in error (being increasingly too large), while formula (1) is not subject to error to such a large degree. Both of course imply a rounded sore as the term 'PI' is involved as a scaler. As an example of a case which is certainly not round, consider a rectangular sore of 10 cm by 0.5 cm (say a surgical wound).

Then, if PI is taken as 3.142 (to 3 decimal places):

Equation (1) gives PI * 5 * 0.25 = 3.627 cm^2.
Equation (2) gives PI * (10 + 0.5)/2 squared or
PI * 5.25 * 5.25 = 95.046 cm^2.

The actual area should be (for a rectangle) one side times the side perpendicular to it, i.e.

Calculated area = 10 * 0.5 = 5 cm^2.

Thus it can be seen that formula (1) actually under-represents the area, but it is only in error by about 28 per cent, but (2) is too high by 1900 per cent, or a factor of 19.

Rhodes *et al.* used the area in a 'healing index', which was:

Healing index = (initial area − final area)/time in days, where area was calculated using formula (1). So this index gives the rate of healing in cm^2 day.

Measurement of area directly

In order to measure shapes that are not uniform, a tracing technique has been used. A variety of materials may be used ranging from old X-ray film, disposable plastic gloves or any transparent medium. This method was used by Taylor *et al.* (1974). No figures for accuracy were given for the readings.

Once the tracing has been taken the area within the tracing can be ascertained by placing over graph paper, or calculated with a planimeter (a device for measuring irregular areas). The planimeter requires a flat surface, hence it may not be used directly on sore surfaces, quite apart from the practical difficulty in so doing. If the planimeter or other method of area calculation is extremely accurate, one may be misled to attribute an inappropriately high level of accuracy to the technique as a whole, for the initial tracing of the sore is subject to large error, as is shown later.

Photography as a method of recording the progress of sores seems intuitively an excellent method as it provides a permanent record and successive pictures may show improvement or deterioration. If there were a fixed distance between the subject and the camera, then in principle a measure could be made. However, unless the photograph is larger than life, no obvious advantage over directly measuring the sore would be obtained. Further there may be some distortion due to different perspective, if successive photographs were taken from slightly different angles. It may be useful to photograph for quite different reasons, such as showing the patient the sore if they are unable by virtue of its position to see it. This may be very useful to achieve patient compliance in treatment, and to show continuous improvement thus maintaining morale. But as a measuring technique photography is fraught with problems.

Taylor *et al.* (1974) tried to overcome the problems involved in photography by photographing from a plane perpendicular to the axis of the sore, with a centimetre circle as a standard, placed next to the sore when it was photographed. The slide produced was enlarged onto graph paper, and the squares counted both in the tracing of the sore and of the standard circle. Thus the area may be computed. Despite this sophistication, Taylor *et al.* stated that the images traced directly were more reliable.

Measurement of volume

Measurement of one length produces a one-dimensional result. Measurement of two lengths produces a two-dimensional result, which is expressed as an area. But sores, like all real objects are three-dimensional. It is true that many superficial sores are adequately modelled as two-dimensional structures, but ideally sores would be represented in three dimensions. This is particularly pertinent for cavernous sores. A sore which is healing from the base up will not necessarily appear to heal if area alone is calculated.

Woodbine (1979) describes sores as having two lengths and depth. She does not state what criteria were used to determine the lengths, or the depth. It would be logical to measure the deepest point of a sore, as the sore graduates from this point to the skin surface continuously, and any other criterion would be difficult to define. She gives depths to one decimal place of a centimetre. There is more difficulty in measuring depth than diameters, as one would need to look at the ruler perpendicular to the plane of the sore, and take the line of the sore edge as the position on the ruler to read from. The above assumes a ruler was used, unless some more sophisticated technique were employed it seems unlikely that such a high level of accuracy can be achieved. No estimate is given of error in this study.

A method developed at the Geriatric Research Unit at St Pancras Hospital (Cottenden, 1986) attempts to determine depth not just at one point, but in a variety of points. A set of rounded metal pins which are freely mobile in a Perspex holder are lowered into the sore, where they rest on the sore-bed. They thus form a contour of the sore. The pins are clamped at this juncture and then the apparatus is lifted out. This method will not necessarily take the deepest point of the sore, but if a sufficient number of pins are used a repeatable result should be obtained. The pins may be numbered, and the pins touching the healthy skin around the sore may be noted. Then one may manually or automatically measure the relative distance between the sore edge and any point where a pin rests on the sore bed. This measurement could be achieved via a calibrated set of marks on the instrument, or by electrical signals being fed into a microcomputer from the apparatus. Alternatively the profile of pins could be traced onto graph paper, the two pins first to rest on healthy skin outside the sore could be taken as zero, a straight line drawn between them on the graph paper, allowing the depth of each point to be directly read from accurately calibrated paper. The cross-sectional area may be measured by counting squares inside the tracing and the line drawn. If the pins are close together the several lines joining the pin-heads approximate the curve of the wound bed. One or more such profiles could be used as the basis for calculating volume of the sore. Sores with large radii of curvature will be under-represented by this method, as a drawn straight line will lie beneath the actual curve of the sore.

There will be the same problem then as in the case for devising formulae that accurately calculate area based on one or more diameters, which is that the formulae may become increasingly inaccurate for extreme shapes. The greater the number of profiles (i.e. the more the data), the more certain of accuracy we may be. However, there is a problem of ascertaining the distance between the profiles, and of maintaining the axes of the successive profiles parallel to each other. A calibrated frame could house the 'profilometer' much as an X-ray machine, or a telescope mounting maintains a fixed plane. This does assume the patient does not move between measurements, which must be likely in confused or debilitated patients. To overcome this problem there could be an array of pins, consisting of several rows, which may be employed to take several profiles simultaneously.

At present the 'profilometer' has been tested as a prototype, where one profile is taken, and measured manually. No assessments of accuracy have been done, but a maximum expected accuracy would probably be in the order of a millimetre.

Pories *et al.* (1966) measured wounds following excision of pilonidal sinuses. Their method employed an alginate hydrocolloid (Jeltrate) as used in dental work. This material, which is a rapidly setting plastic was used to make an impression of the wound.

The volumetric measurements were then produced by placing the impressions in a graduated cylinder part filled with water. The volume displaced by the impression would be seen as a rise of water in the cylinder.

The difficulty of this technique is in producing a surface of the impression flush with the sore edges. In deep sores with a relatively small cross-sectional area, such as post pilo-nidal sinus surgery this may not generate a large error. But in many decubitus ulcers the ratio of length to depth may be quite large, and varicose ulcers almost invariably have a high ratio. Any error in the vertical plane would give rise to large error. No mention of error is given by Pories *et al.* in their study. But the sores were noted to heal in this particular case logarithmically, i.e. the healing was fast to start with, and decelerated. What error there is becomes increasingly relevant as the sore is reduced in size. Alternatively the rapid initial healing was measured with greater accuracy than the final stage close to healing.

This is quite satisfactory when measuring an acute condition like surgical wounds in young patients, with logarithmic healing. It presents with more difficulty in indolent sores such as decubitus ulcers and varicose ulcers. This is because these sores heal over periods of months, averaging about four months, and may increase in size, rather than heal. Further the normal healing process in decubitus ulcers, and the healing of indolent sores show a linear pattern against time in contrast to acute wounds described above (Barton and Barton, 1973). Thus the 'healing index' as described by Rhodes will usually be a constant in these sores.

Tomography

Computed tomography has been used to assess pressure sores. Firooznia et al. (1983) stated that the technique gave 'the exact size, depth, and degree of undermining of the edge' of pressure sores. No values for these measures were given in their study, nor of accuracy. They note that small sore openings often hide much larger lesions in deep sores, and this is a method which is suitable for such cases. In 36 sores on 23 patients with spinal cord injury, tomography revealed the size and undermining of 34 sores. Four sores with small openings had extensive undermining, four extended into the hip joint, four had associated fistulae as found by tomography, fourteen had soft tissue abscesses, five of which had not been clinically recognized, and fourteen cases of osteomyelitis were identified. Sinus tracts which occur in 10–15 per cent of spinal cord patients with grade III or IV pressure sores were also identifiable by this technique. Whatever one interprets as 'exact' for its measures of size and depth, this is clearly a technique with much promise in the diagnosis of complications of sores, and in pre-operative planning of surgical repair of deep sores.

Stereophotogrammetry

This method has been used to measure area, volume and wound edge length (Gunnel Erickson et al., 1979). Two cameras take photographs simultaneously, these are then analysed using a stereocomparator. This instrument creates a three-dimensional image by combining the two images created by the photographs. A 'measuring mark' may be mechanically moved around the image, and three-dimensional coordinates may be read from the instrument. By superimposing this mark on various points of the image of the sore, a profile of the sore may be built up.

By taking points around the sore edge, the sore edge length may be determined, area may be computed using a formula that is discussed later in the next section of this chapter (equation (4)). Volume may be determined by taking profiles as described above for the profilometer. Diameters can also be calculated if wished.

The accuracy of the equipment is reported as 1 micrometre for the stereocomparator. The total apparatus is calculated to give absolute errors of 0.2 mm in depth, and less in the horizontal components. This is said to result in approximately 0.03 mm error for wound edge length, 5 mm^2 for area and 35 mm^2 for volume. The error introduced by the observer in delineating the true edge of the sore is an order of magnitude higher than this. Gunnel Eriksson et al. repeated one observation and found a difference of 2.3 mm in wound length, 30.9 mm^2 for area and 65.3 mm^3 for volume from a sore with average reading of edge length 85 mm, area 530 mm^2 and volume 700 mm.[3]

This method appears to give accurate measurement of all the dimensions, and is a non-contact method. However, one needs a stereocomparator and two high quality cameras need to be specially modified and placed accurately on a rigid bar. So for routine clinical work, or multicentre trials it will be prohibitively expensive. The points measured with the stereocomparator are measured manually by an operator, and an increase in sore definition requires greater time and effort.

The Computer-aided Method

A computer-aided method was developed in which a photographic slide of a sore, with a known area surrounding it is projected or enlarged onto a digitizer. The image of the sore and the standard area are traced with a probe, the area being calculated by a microcomputer (Anthony and Barnes, 1984).

Photography as previously mentioned is not without its difficulties. Rather than use a range of set distances from which to photograph the sore, or calculate the perspective correction after measuring the distance between camera and subject, a relative approach was chosen. A known area was placed close to the sore. Thus a scaling factor is introduced. This is a slightly more sophisticated version of placing a coin next to a photographed object. Originally a one centimetre circle was placed next to the sore, but the errors obtained in tracing such a small area were unacceptable (about 50 per cent for large sores, the error increasing paradoxically with larger sores, as the circle appears smaller in the photograph. This is the same problem presumably that Taylor et al. (1974) encountered. So a frame was made of polyester, with an accurately marked grid printed on it. This allowed frames a little larger than the sore under consideration. A nest of regular figures were used, a close fit being applied to any particular sore.

The images of sore and frame may be traced manually onto graph paper, but this is tedious and slow. The computer allows semi-automatic computation of these areas using a similar trace technique with an electronically read probe.

Photographic slide film was used, though photographic enlargement could produce a similar, but more expensive result. The slide of a sore and frame was enlarged onto the measuring apparatus, to reduce error in tracing. A vertically mounted slide-projector could be used for this purpose, but a photographic enlarger was used, as it is mounted vertically already. This necessitated a dark-room.

A BBC Model B microcomputer was connected to a digitizer via the analogue port of the computer. A digitizer is an instrument for transforming an input which may have any value in a continuous range of values (i.e. an analogue value — an example is length, where an item's length may be any number in principle) into a digital output. A digital output is one which may only take one of a limited number of values — an example would be the number of people in a family, for there may be one, two, three, but not 2.7. The limited range which describes family size is composed of the natural (counting) numbers, which excludes decimals and fractions. The input from the digitizer is a voltage, which is analogue. Except for some large computers, only digital values may be processed by a computer, hence the need for digitization. One may understand this as a consequence of the method of the sending information to the microprocessor, which is by electronic pulses. Sending a pulse means one, not sending it is zero. The writing of a computer program consists in its most elemental level, of essentially sending yes or no, 1 or 0. This is the simplest possible case of a digital system (excluding the trivial case of a system with only one state or only one number, which is not a system capable of sending information since it will always say the same thing), and being a system with two states, or numerals, is called binary.

The digitizer is the apparatus chosen to feed information to the computer, to enable it to measure an area. A probe is attached to a board with a grid marked on it, by a Perspex arm jointed in two places to allow it to move to any point in a horizontal plane. At the centre of each hinge lies a potentiometer, which is a device for changing voltage (a common example is the volume dial of a transistor radio). As the hinge turns the voltage output by the digitizer is altered. Two separate voltages, one from each potentiometer, are fed from the digitizer to the computer, through the analogue port (a port is simply a physical point of entry for voltage input/output of the computer). These two inputs 'tell' the computer where the probe is. This is made simpler as the digitizer is designed to give an output voltage from the potentiometers that are directly proportional to the angles the hinges are turned through. That is, there is a linear relationship between angle turned and voltage.

The point on any plane may be found by simple trigonometry, if the two angles of the Perspex arm holding the probe are ascertained. The details of this relationship are contained in Appendix 1. This will need to be read by potential users of this system if they use any digitizer other than the PL digitizer.

If the coordinates of the probe are found by the above method, an area can be calculated. This is done by the following algorithm (Linney, 1984):

For two consecutive points with coordinates x_1, y_1 and x_2, y_2 respectively, the area under a line joining these points is:

$$\text{Area} = (x_2 - x_1) * (y_1 + y_2)/2 \qquad (4)$$

For many points along a line, the area may be approximated to the sum of several areas under successive point pairs. Whichever way the sore is traced the effect of the algorithm is to compute the area closed in by curve. For the lower portion of the curve is traced right to left if the upper is traced left to right and vice versa. Therefore on tracing the lower curve clockwise $x_2 < x_1$ always thus producing a negative area to deduct from a positive value for the area under the top portion. If the curve is traced anti-clockwise the areas are still opposite in sign, the final result will be negative rather than positive, but the same absolute value. Since negative areas do not interest us, being merely information as to the direction of the tracing, the algorithm is understood to output only positive values, negative ones have their sign changed.

There is an approximation inherent in the calculation as the curve will be inaccurately represented by straight lines joining the points. However, if sufficient points are considered one may achieve as high a degree of accuracy as required. There is some fluctuation in the voltage even if the probe is stationary, due to random small changes in the voltage from factors other than the probe's movement. It is sensible to consider the accuracy in the range of the capability of the digitizer in differentiating voltages. This was achieved by allowing the computer to read the position of the probe continuously while it was kept static, and to print a result only if the new plot was found to be different by a given amount than the original plot. This amount was gradually made smaller until a point was reached when the difference was smaller than the randomness inherent in the system. This was found to occur at a voltage difference equivalent to 1/1000 of the maximum length the board allows measurement of. At twice this value, the probe registered as stable in position if left for several minutes. Below this level, areas may be output even if the probe is not moved. This error will become increasingly apparent as the distance allowed before a point is considered different from a prior plot, is decreased. Since the errors are likely to be random, and will tend to cancel each other out, due to the effect described above of anti-clockwise and clockwise having opposite signs, this error is important for small sores only. The program design allows new points to be plotted only when a distance greater than 2/1000 of the size of the board was registered as an equivalent voltage difference.

The Program

The program used for pressure sore measurement, which is included as Appendix 2, is divided into several parts:

(1) The digitizer is calibrated by the operator placing the probe on preselected positions.
(2) The textural data to be displayed in the print-out is input (name of patient, date, etc.).
(3) The number of repeat measurements wanted is input, with the size of frame used as a standard to compare with the tracing of the sore.
(4) The sore image is traced several times, each tracing is accompanied with a tracing of the standard area. The sore tracing is displayed on the monitor, so one may check that the sore has been traced back to its starting point. At any time a tracing may be aborted, thus accidental errors due to slips of the hand may be eliminated. The areas and coordinates of the probe are not printed out until all the tracings have been completed, thus one may not be biased to try to get similar results, other than by accurately tracing the area.

(5) The areas are analysed simply by mean and standard deviation.
(6) The results and textural information are printed out both to screen and printer, a hard copy is thus obtained.

Comparisons of Several Methods

Bohannon and Pfaller (1983) compared three methods of measuring:

(1) Tracing with a transparent medium followed by placing the tracing over metric graph paper and counting squares within the shape.
(2) Using planimetry of such a tracing, and
(3) Weighing a cut-out shape of a tracing on accurate scales.

They assessed the highest possible accuracy of each technique by drawing known circular areas onto graph paper, and counting squares, by tracing a known circular area with the planimeter, and by weighing four known squares, dividing by the total known area to get a weight per unit area, and using this to calculate the four individual areas. In all cases very high levels of accuracy were obtained, always <1.2 per cent from the known area.

Two clinicians measured five sores on three patients on the same day. Additionally two sores were traced by each on two different days, and one sore by each on three different days.

The mean differences in values between the observers was 4.4, 3.9 and 3.6 per cent for the weighing, tracing and planimetry methods, respectively.

The authors concluded that the difficulty in delineating the wound edge caused the greater error on actual wounds compared with known areas.

Anthony (1985) compared the tracing method with the computer-aided method and measurement of longest and shortest diameters.

The digitizer–computer system has been tested for accuracy on known irregular shapes of various sizes and contours, photographed in a plane and distorted on pliable card (Barnes et al., 1984). The accuracy in area was generally in the order of 2 per cent. In order to discover whether the computer method was in practice as accurate as these bench tests showed it to be, it was tested on a small sample of sores. In addition the common methods of tracing longest and shortest diameters were compared with the computer method. (The same sores were used on the same days for each method.)

Procedure

Three observers each measured a sore ten times on the same day as each other, and each sore was measured by the three techniques.

Results

The results are summarized in Tables 1 to 4.

Two types of comparison may obviously be made.

One observer may measure a particular sore slightly differently each time, giving rise to inter-observer variability. This variability was higher in all cases for the computer-aided method, than the variability noted in bench tests discussed above. The variability was higher still with the other two methods, the highest variability was noted for the trace method.

Table 1 Measurements by computer-aided method. Reproduced by permission of *Nursing Times*

Subject A	Measurer 1 ($n = 10$)	Measurer 2 ($n = 10$)	Measurer 3 ($n = 10$)
Mean	18.91	18.81	20.40
SD/Mean %	4.4	2.8	9.0

No significant difference between means.

Subject B	Measurer 1 ($n = 10$)	Measurer 2 ($n = 10$)	Measurer 3 ($n = 10$)
Mean	1.29	1.10	0.95
SD/Mean %	7.0	4.5	8.4

Significant difference between means ($p < 0.01$).

Subject C	Measurer 1 ($n = 10$)	Measurer 2 ($n = 10$)	Measurer 3 ($n = 10$)
Mean	1.29	1.74	1.23
SD/Mean %	12.4	28.2	24.4

No significant difference between means.

Subject D	Measurer 1 ($n = 10$)	Measurer 2 ($n = 10$)	Measurer 3 ($n = 10$)
Mean	2.17	2.29	2.94
SD/Mean %	5.5	16.2	9.5

Significant difference between means ($p < 0.01$).

Table 2   Measurements by trace method. Reproduced by permission of
Nursing Times

Subject A	Measurer 1 (n = 10)	Measurer 2 (n = 10)	Measurer 3 (n = 10)
Mean	14.34	15.22	16.47
SD/Mean %	15.4	12.3	16.1

No significant difference between means.

Subject B	Measurer 1 (n = 10)	Measurer 2 (n = 10)	Measurer 3 (n = 10)
Mean	1.00	0.95	0.66
SD/Mean %	10.0	17.9	12.1

Significant difference between means ($p < 0.01$).

Subject C	Measurer 1 (n = 6)	Measurer 2 (n = 6)	Measurer 3 (n = 6)
Mean	0.61	1.19	1.05
SD/Mean %	42.6	10.1	20.9

Significant difference between means ($p < 0.01$).

Subject D	Measurer 1 (n = 10)	Measurer 2 (n = 10)	Measurer 3 (n = 10)
Mean	2.50	5.01	7.49
SD/Mean %	29.8	17.0	13.1

Significant difference between means ($p < 0.01$).

Table 3   Measurements by longest diameter. Reproduced by permission of
Nursing Times

Subject A	Measurer 1 (n = 10)	Measurer 2 (n = 10)	Measurer 3 (n = 10)
Mean	8.19	7.75	6.87
SD/Mean %	2.1	2.1	4.7

Significant difference between means ($p < 0.01$).

Subject B	Measurer 1 (n = 10)	Measurer 2 (n = 10)	Measurer 3 (n = 10)
Mean	1.93	1.76	1.53
SD/Mean %	4.7	6.8	4.6

Significant difference between means ($p < 0.01$).

Table 4   Measurements by shortest diameter. Reproduced by permission of *Nursing Times*

Subject A	Measurer 1 (n = 10)	Measurer 2 (n = 10)	Measurer 3 (n = 10)
Mean	1.45	1.94	1.82
SD/Mean %	11.0	4.1	11.0

Significant difference between means ($p < 0.01$).

Subject B	Measurer 1 (n = 10)	Measurer 2 (n = 10)	Measurer 3 (n = 10)
Mean	1.30	1.45	1.63
SD/Mean %	6.2	5.5	4.3

Significant difference between means ($p < 0.01$).

For any particular method of measurement, one may compare the values obtained by different observers. This between observer variability may be used in conjunction with the inter-observer variability, to determine whether the mean values obtained are significantly different from each other. For the four sores measured, two were significantly different as measured by different observers, for the computer-aided method, three of the four sores measured by the trace method and all four measurements taken on the two sores by the diameter method were significantly different.

Discussion

On a small sample of four sores, the computer method was most consistent both inter-observer and between observers. Surprisingly the tracing method fared worse than longest and shortest diameters with regard to inter-observer error. This would indicate that the easier method of longest and shortest diameters is more repeatable than tracing, provided that the same observer is used.

One has to be cautious when comparing the measurements of diameters with the other two methods for two reasons:

(1) The diameter method was only employed on two sores, not on all four.
(2) The tracings measure area directly. Diameters measure only length, and to obtain an approximate area one has to use one of the formulae mentioned above (equations (1) and (2)). To do this

requires both longest and shortest diameters, so the errors should
be added for the longest and shortest diameters.

To easily compare the errors of the different sores one may compute
the standard deviation/mean. In this study it was expressed as a
percentage.

If the errors for diameters are added, and only sores measured by
all three methods are used the mean of this value are:

Computer method   6.0 per cent
Trace method   14.0 per cent
Diameter method   11.4 per cent

The variance of a particular observer in repeated measurements is to
be expected, as the analogue nature of the sore area would require
infinite accuracy for full repeatability to be achieved. The question is
not whether variance will occur, but how much variance there will be.

One would expect that different people would get similar readings
for the same sore. This was found not to be the case in two of four of
the computer measurements, three of four of the tracings, and all of
the diameters, using the analysis of variance as a criterion. It would be
bold to put the techniques in a ranked order of preference on these
findings, as the sample is small. But it would appear that different
people actually are measuring different sores. This is due, presumably,
to different criteria being employed to determine the edge of the sore.
There is an additional problem with the tracing technique, in that the
sore is partially obscured by the medium on which it is be drawn, and
the pen used will be drawn on the outside, or the inside of the sore
edge, giving different readings in each case.

Sources of Error in Measurement

The following section describes errors that may be encountered in many
areas of measurement, not just pressure sores.

Accuracy of the Instrument Used

In this case we are considering a physical instrument. There are always
limits imposed by the apparatus itself. The accuracy of the instrument
should be such as to make meaningful analysis possible. The ruler has
calibrated marks, and anything smaller than those calibrations can not
be accurately measured, although one may take a rough guess (an

object that apparently covers about half the distance between two calibrated points may be said to be about half a 'calibration length' long).

It might be thought that increasing the number of calibration points will improve accuracy, but there is a limit to how near they may be, and still be seen by the human eye. Since the human observer is a part of the apparatus in a ruler measurement, there is no point in going below this limit. One would not use a ruler to measure the distance between atoms. More generally a system of measurement is only as good as its weakest link.

So the accuracy is set at that level, and further improvement will first look to the weakest component. Very small distances of the order of individual cells for example, must be achieved with a more powerful technique like microscopy. Eventually light is insufficient to be used at subcellular distances, as its resolving power becomes a limiting factor. This is analogous to using a yard rule to measure the width of a human hair, it is too large an instrument. Electron beams may be used in an electron microscope for very small objects. At atomic levels even electrons are too big, and a technique known as X-ray crystallography is employed.

At the other extreme a method may be too sensitive or unnecessarily accurate. One does not need to know the size of a football pitch to millionths of a centimetre, in any event getting it under the electron microscope presents with technical difficulties!

The Instrument's Effect on the Parameter

Sometimes the fact that a situation is being measured can change that situation, so it ceases to be was to be measured. This may be the cause of artefacts in electron microscopy, as only dead tissue can be analysed, which is then specially treated, so the item viewed may be very different from the living untreated material. Another example would be blood pressure monitoring. Simply by recording it, one may induce anxiety and raise blood pressure, which will result in an over-estimate. These problems are at least as problematic in sociological type instruments. For the way a subject answers a question will depend to some extent on the way it is asked, whether in writing or by a researcher talking to them, by the language used, and by in the latter case intonation and manner.

It might be thought that given sufficient resources one may always reach perfect accuracy. It is thought by most theoretical physicists that even in simple physical measurement this is not true, there is a theoretical limit as well as a practical limit, to what may be achieved.

The Calculation as a Source of Error

If some theoretical argument is used to derive or calculate from even perfectly accurate data, error will be input potentially by the calculation. Thus in the example of calculating areas by using a modified formula for a circle's area on non-circular areas, error will become obvious for some shapes. In a questionnaire determining whether a subject is extravert, if the questions are badly chosen, so they do not correctly pick out extravert attitudes, even a scrupulously honest filling in of a questionnaire will give misleading results.

In computers, and calculators, which work to a set number of decimal points, 'rounding errors' will be introduced as numbers are represented by the nearest number that the machine may allocate. This error must be borne in mind even if the machine works to a much higher degree of accuracy than the final result need be expressed in. For if certain manipulations are done, huge errors may accrue. An example would be where one number is subtracted from another. If the numbers are very similar, and if the result is used in division or multiplication later in the calculation, an error such as in the example below may occur.

A micrometer accurate to 0.01 of a millimetre is used to measure two lengths, and the difference between the lengths is required. Assume one length (say length 1) is 1.004 mm and the other is 1.006 mm (length 2).

If the micrometer records the lengths as 1.00 and 1.01 respectively then:

inaccuracy of length 1 is $100 * (1.004 - 1.000)/1.004$ = approx. 0.4 per cent
inaccuracy of length 2 is $100 * (1.010 - 1.006)/1.006$ = approx. 0.4 per cent

The difference between the lengths is actually $1.006 - 1.004 = 0.002$ mm
But it is measured as $1.01 - 1.00 = 0.01$ mm. The inaccuracy in the difference is:

$100 * 0.01/0.002$ per cent = 500 per cent

Thus the measurement of the difference is proportionately inaccurate compared with the real difference in the original lengths. It is reasonable to state that the absolute accuracy is the same, namely 0.01 mm, and the inaccuracy reported is an artefact caused by the way we have chosen to represent it, as a percentage. This is true, however, if the difference is used as a divisor or multiplier in subsequent expressions or analysis this error will be passed on in full, however large the other numbers involved may be, and despite great accuracy in their measurement.

This is an example of a phenomenon, called 'numerical instability'. It can be minimized by a variety of techniques known collectively as 'numerical analysis'.

Referring back to the equation used in computing area (equation (4)) it would appear we have this problem, as the difference of two x axis coordinates is multiplied by the average of two y coordinates. Any small error in an x value will greatly affect the value for area.

Suppose that in computing a series of areas from the x coordinates x_1, x_2, x_3, x_4, etc. (where $x_4 > x_3 > x_2 > x_1$) the x_2 coordinate is overestimated, then $x_2 - x_1$ will be larger than it should be, returning a higher area than it should. But then the next area $x_3 - x_2$ will be too small by the same amount. Since the average of the y coordinates is changing relatively slowly for small increments of x, the error is almost totally cancelled over successive elemental area additions. Thus what appears to be a classic case of numerical instability is in fact quite well behaved.

Conclusion

Despite the apparent triviality of the problem of measuring a sore, there turns out to be many complications if an accurate and repeatable result is needed. This is probably more important in research than in clinical practice, as the accurate methods described above are too time consuming to be used routinely. But if sores are to be measured as clinical indicators, it is well to be aware of the likely error bounds. Even for many repeated measurements with a mean value computed, one must accept an error of 10–20 per cent as minimum, for the tracing and ruler approaches. Using more than one measurer seems to be associated with further error, as different people delineate different sore edges, or get statistically different areas by some other mechanism.

Any improvement in accuracy of measurement achieved by better equipment will be overshadowed by the weakest part of the apparatus, the human interpretation of sore boundary. A way automatically to compute area from an image of a sore would be to digitize the information from a video-camera into a microcomputer, and use changes in intensity of reflected light or colour to be accepted as boundaries. Software and camera equipment already exist which can do this. One would need to establish only that what the software computes as an area relates to what is perceived as a sore. The result might not be more accurate, but it would be more repeatable. In principle such an approach could be applied to the three-dimensional images of stereo-photogrammery, though the algorithms will be more complex.

Acknowledgements

Grateful thanks to: Elizabeth Barnes, Professor A. N. Exton-Smith, Alf Linney, James Malone-Lee and Janet Simpson. Illustration by Michael Mooney.

References

Anthony, D. (1985). Measuring pressure sores. *Nursing Times*, 29 May, **81** (22), 57–61.
Anthony, D. and Barnes, E. (1984). Measuring pressure sores accurately. *Nursing Times*, 5 Sept, **80** (36), 33–35.
Barton, A. A. and Barton, M. (1973). The clinical and thermographical evaluation of pressure sores. *Age and Aging*, **2** (55), 55–59.
Barnes, E., Anthony, D., Exton-Smith, E. N. and Malone-Lee, J. (1984). *An Accurate Method of Measuring Pressure Sores*. Paper presented to Society for Tissue Viability.
Barnes, E. and Malone-Lee, J. (1985). Tegaderm pouch dressings. *Nursing Times*, 27 Nov., **81** (48), 45–46.
Bohannon, R. W. and Pfaller, B. A. (1983). Documentation of wound surface area from tracings of wound perimeters. *Physical Therapy*, Oct., **63** (10), 1622–1624.
Cottenden, A. (1986). Personal communication.
David, J. (1984). Tissue breakdown. *Nursing Times*, 7 March, **158** (10), Clinical Forum, i–x.
Firooznia, H., Mahvash, R., Golimbu, C. and Sokolow, J. (1983). Computed tomography of pressure sores. *The Journal of Computed Tomography*, **7** (4), 367–373.
Gunnel Erikson, Eklund, A. E., Torlegard, K. and Dauphin E. (1979). Evaluation of leg ulcer treatment with stereogrammetry. *British Journal of Dermatology*, **101** (123), 123–131.
Linney, A. (1984). Personal communication.
Pories, W. J., Schear, E. W., Jordan, D. R., Chase, J., Parkinson, G., Whittaker, R. Strain, W. H. and Rob, C. (1966). The measurement of human wound healing. *Surgery*, May, **59** (5), 821–824.
Rhodes, B., Daltrey, D., Chattwood, J. G. (1979). The treatment of pressure sores in geriatric patients. *Nursing Times*, 1 March, **75** (9), 365–368.
Taylor, T. J., Rimmer, S., Day, B., Butcher, J. and Dymock, I. W. (1974).

Ascorbic acid supplementation in the treatment of pressure sores. *The Lancet*, 7 Sept, 544–546.

Waterlow (1985). A Risk Assessment Card. *Nursing Times*, 27 Nov., **81** (48), 49–55.

Woodbine, A. (1979). A survey in Macclesfield. *Nursing Times*, 5 July, **75** (27), 1128–1132.

Appendix 1: Configuration of PL Digitizer

Figure 1 shows the configuration of the PL digitizer. 'A' is the angle between the top arm of the digitizer, which is fixed to the board, and the vertical. 'B' is the angle between the fixed arm and the free arm. All angles are expressed in degrees here.

angle EAB = A
angle ABC = B

then:

$$\text{angle ABE} = (90 - A)$$

therefore angle $EBC = B - (90 - A)$

$$\text{angle DBC} = 90 - [B - (90 - A)]$$
$$= 180 - (A + B)$$

If the fixed arm is of length L_1, and the free arm of length L_2, then:

$$xx = L_1 * \sin(A) - L_2 * \sin[180 - (A + B)]$$
$$yy = L_2 * \cos(A) - L_2 * \cos[180 - (A + B)]$$

Where xx and yy are horizontal and vertical distances respectively from the fixed hinge.

It can be shown that:

$$\sin(180\text{-angle}) = + \sin(\text{angle})$$
$$\text{and } \cos(180\text{-angle}) = - \cos(\text{angle})$$

so:

$$xx = L_1 * \sin(A) - L_2 * \sin(A + B)$$
$$yy = L_1 * \cos(A) - L_2 * [- \cos(A + B)] \text{ or}$$
$$yy = L_1 * \cos(A) + L_2 * \cos(A + B)$$

But it is also a property of sine and cosine that:

$$\sin(\text{-angle}) = - \sin(\text{angle})$$
$$\text{and } \cos(\text{-angle}) = \cos(\text{angle})$$

so:

$$xx = L_1 * \sin(A) + L_2 * \sin(A + B)$$
$$yy = L_1 * \cos(A) + L_2 * \cos(A + B)$$

If you look at lines 240 and 250 of the computer program, the above expressions have been used. Though the actual lengths are entered (28 and 18 cm) and the expressions have been divided through by L_2.

Also note line 80 where the angles TA, PA are the angles 'A' and 'B' above,

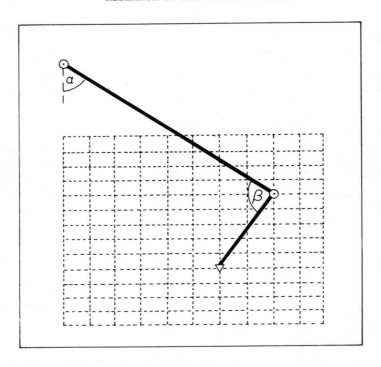

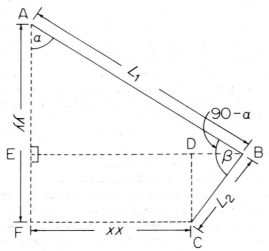

Figure 1   Geometry of digitizer

measured at one calibration point, and TB, PB are the angles at a separate calibration point. These are the points asked for in lines 130 and 150 respectively. They may be any points for which the angles 'A' and 'B' have been measured, but the further apart they are in x and y coordinates, the less the potential error.

If the actual origin from where we measure is different from the fixed hinge, by C_1 in the X axis, and C_2 in the y axis, then:

$$xx = C_1 + L_1 * \sin (A) + L_2* \sin (A + B)$$
$$yy = C_2 + L_2 * \cos (A) + L_2 * \cos (A + B)$$

This correction is not actually necessary for measuring areas, but will be necessary to determine position absolutely.

For a linear relation of voltage to angle, which a good digitizer should allow, line 280 in the program gives the values x and y which are values of voltages from which the angles that the hinges are turned through are derived in line 420.

Appendix 2: BBC Basic Program to Interface Digitizer

```
10AA=-1
20MODE 4
30C$='TO CONTINUE PRESS SPACE BAR'
40S$='TO STOP PRESS SPACE BAR'
50P$='PRESS SPACE BAR'
60CLS
70AREA=0:AR=0
80TA=RAD(128.263921):PA=RAD(20.852708):TB=RAD
(72.7913179):PB=RAD(111.984893):XD=1000:YD=-1000
90A=1:B=1:X0=0:Y0=?:PROCc(TA,PA):XA=XX:YA=YY:PROCc
(TB,PB):XX:YB=YY:A=XD/(XB-XA):B=YD/(YB-YA)
100PROCc(TA,PA):X0=XX:PROCc(TB,PB):Y0=YY
110PRINT`A=';A;`B=';B
120PRINT`X0=';X0;`Y0=';Y0
130PRINT`PLACE PROBE AT TOP LEFT HAND CORNER OF
GRID',P$
140PRINT`POINT A':CX=GET:PROCa:X1=X:Y1=Y
150PRINT`PLACE PROBE AT BOTTOM RIGHT CORNER OF
GRID',P$
160PRINT`POINT B':CX=GET:PROCa:X2=X:Y2=Y
170DIMX(500),Y(500),A(500)
180PROCDATA
190PROCLINK
200 PROCSTATS
210PROCPRINT
220END
230DEFPROCc(T1,T2)
240XX=A*SIN(T1)-A*28/18*SIN(T2+T1)-X0
250YY=B*COS(T1)-B*28/18*COS (T2+T1)-Y0
```

```
260ENDPROC
270DEFPROCa
280X=0:Y=0:FORI=1TO10:X=X+ADVALI:Y=Y+ADVAL2:NEXT:
X=X/10:Y=Y/10
290ENDPROC
300DEFPROCDATA
310CLS
320INPUT'NAME',N$,'DATE',D$,'FRAME AREA',F,'NUMBER OF
REPEATS',R
330ENDPROC
340DEFPROCTRACE
350AREA=0:AR=0:Q%=0
360IFAA>0PRINT'TRACE FRAME'
370IFAA<0PRINT'TRACE ULCER'
380CX=GET
390CLS
400Q%=Q%+1
410PROCa
420T1=TA+(TB-TA)*(X-X1)/(X2-X1):T2=PA+(PB-PA)*
(Y-Y1)/(Y2-Y1)
430PROCc(T1,T2)
440X(Q%)=XX:Y(Q%)=YY
450IFQ%=1THENGOTO400
460Z=INKEY(1)
470IFZ=32THENENDPROC
480IFZ=48THENGOTO350
490IFABS(Y(Q%)-Y(Q%-1))<2THENGOTO410
500IFABS(X(Q%)-X(Q%-1))<2THENGOTO410
510PROCDRAW
520AR=.5*(Y(Q%)+Y(Q%-1))*(X(Q%)-1))
530AREA=AREA+AR
540GOTO400
550ENDPROC
560DEFPROCLINK
570FORJ%=1TOR
575PRINTJ%
580AA=-AA
590PROCTRACE
600PRINT
610FR=AREA
620AA=-AA
630PROCTRACE
640A(J%)=ABS((AREA/FR)*F)
650PRINT
660NE%TJ%
670ENDPROC
680DEFPROCPRINT
690VDU2
700PRINT'NAME',N$
```

```
710PRINT'DATE',D$
720PRINT'FRAME AREA =',F
730PRINT
760FORK%=1TOR
770PRINTA(K%)
780NEXTK%
790PRINT
800PRINT'STANDARD DEVIATION=',S
810PRINT
860VDU3
870ENDPROC
880DEFPROCSTATS
890A=0:S=0
900FORJ%=1TOR
910A=A+(J%)
920NEXTJ%
930A=A/R
940FORJ%=1TOR
950SD=(A(J%)-A)^2
960S=S+SD
970NEXTJ%
980S=(S/(R-1))^.5
990P=2*S/A
1000ENDPROC
1010DEFPROCDRAW
1020MOVE(X(Q%-1)*.B+150),(Y(Q%-1)*.8+150)
1030DRAWX(Q%)*.8+150,Y(Q%)*.8+150
1040ENDPROC
```

Research in the Nursing Care of Elderly People
Edited by P. Fielding
© 1987 John Wiley & Sons Ltd

CHAPTER 2

Monitoring Bowel Habit in Elderly People

K. Elizabeth Barnes

Introduction

Constipation is a common problem in the elderly population, with a high number requiring aperients to maintain regular bowel function. It is possible that this may be due to physiological age change, to alterations in diet and life-style or to the long-term laxative usage reported by many elderly people.

Mean intestinal transit time (MTT) has been studied by many methods, including the administration of inert markers or dyes, or of radioactive capsules. However, many of these techniques require a high degree of motivation and co-operation by the subject, frequently involving stool collections over a period of days or even weeks. In the case of elderly in-patients, a great deal of input is also demanded from nursing staff, particularly when patients are demented or too ill to be co-operative.

A simple method of measuring MTT has been used to compare two groups of constipated elderly people taking different aperients. The results of this study, and the advantages and disadvantages of using this method are discussed, and the implications for nurses outlined.

Constipation in the Elderly

Constipation in the elderly is widely reported, and many old people regularly take aperients to maintain a daily bowel action. Frequently this has been a lifelong habit; the custom of 'a bath and a dose of salts' every Friday was well-established in the early part of the century.

However, this habit was rarely maintained in response to true consti-pation as we now understand it. Even as recently as 1937, Hurst defined constipation as a condition in which food residue failed to be excreted within 48 hours of ingestion, a definition few medical practitioners would agree with today. The 'great medical myth' of auto-intoxication was prevalent at that time, with the general opinion of lay people and professionals being that a daily bowel action was necessary to prevent poisoning by the accumulation of waste matter. One has sympathy for the Victorian mother trying to monitor the bowel habits of a large family; it is perhaps unsurprising that regular purgation and bowel-consciousness became so common.

This heavy laxative use has continued so that today's elderly popu-lation are more likely than their younger counterparts to use aperients. Connell *et al.* (1965), found laxative use to increase from 5.6 per cent in the age group 30–39 years, to 30.2 per cent in the age group 60–69. This is the same age cohort who in 1943 were aged 40–49, and found by Parks (1943) to have a laxative usage rate of 28.6 per cent. The laxative usage rate of this group has increased only slightly over the years between Parks's study and that of Connell; a high usage rate has thus been a feature of this group for many years. The evidence of Milne and Williamson (1972) supports this; they studied bowel habits in older people and found 38 per cent of men and 50 per cent of women used laxatives. Again, their conclusion was that older people cling to outmoded ideas popular in their youth, and regard infrequent bowel movements as a sign of ill-health.

It is difficult to determine whether this high laxative usage rate is solely due to habit, or to a real tendency to constipation in old age. Certainly the old appear to complain of constipation more, and it has been said that constipation is the commonest disorder of the gastrointes-tinal tract in old age (Exton-Smith, 1972). However, several studies have produced evidence which seems to deny any general age change in bowel habit.

The Ageing Bowel

Cell turnover is more rapid in the gastrointestinal system than anywhere else in the body. In addition, the bowel has an enormous surface area, and secretes and absorbs large quantities of materials throughout the day. There is active and vigorous motility. All these points indicate that the bowel should be an ideal area for the study of age effects (Bhanthumnavin and Schuster, 1977), but in practice, only scanty evidence is available. This situation is made more difficult by the fact that it is hard, if not impossible to differentiate between age changes and changes due to diseases which are more common in later life.

Physiological Changes

Yamagata (1965) studied age changes in a series comparing biopsy specimens from 222 healthy subjects with autopsy specimens from 160 hospital patients. He noted abnormalities of the intestinal glands, mucosae, an increase in connective tissue, arteriolar sclerosis and atrophy of the muscle layer. Studying the epithelial cells by electron microscopy showed an increased number of small vacuoles, an increase in electron density of the cell, and abnormalities of the nuclei. Mars and Buogo (1967) reported a high incidence of colonic diverticula (47 per cent) in a random series of 104 autopsies from a geriatric institution.

Changes in Bowel Motility

The subject of intestinal motility is an important one for research as diseases and age-associated changes in other systems, for example the nervous system, may show an effect in bowel motility. Again, it is difficult to separate true age effects from disease processes, but there have been some limited studies of gut motility in old age.

Three components of intestinal motility are generally recognized. The first is basal tonus, which refers simply to the inherent amount of contraction in the gut musculature. The second, and most common, is rhythmic segmentation. This occurs in response to many stimuli, and serves to move the food bolus around in the same area of the intestine. Finally, there is propulsive activity whereby the bolus is moved along the gut, sometimes as an effect of systolic contraction, and sometimes as a phased contraction of the muscle. If the distal portion of the gut is relaxed, large boli of faeces may be moved rapidly along substantial lengths of colon, with propulsion aided by postural changes (Connell, 1972). Such mass movements may also be caused by a segmenting wave if it is associated with distal relaxation.

Motility increases during and after ingestion of food. However, the movement is propulsive only in those people who are physically active (Holdstock et al., 1970). The lack of propulsive movements in resting subjects may help to explain the occurrence of constipation in the immobile elderly. Both hypermotility and hypomotility may be associated with the administration of drugs.

The rectum too is associated with rhythmic contractions. Here the contractions are of greater frequency than in the sigmoid, and their frequency increases again nearer the anus (Connell, 1972). This is a continence mechanism designed to hold the bulk of the faeces in the upper rectum. The threshold for recognition of the call to stool decreases as the anus is approached.

Neglect of the Call to Stool

Distension of the rectum can be recognized by normal subjects after instillation of 36 ml of air (Frenckner and Ihre, 1976). They found the maximal tolerable discomfort to be 363 ml. An age change in this mechanism has been reported by Newman and Freeman (1974), who found an increase with age in the volume of rectal distension required to produce discomfort. This was even more marked in constipated subjects.

This age change in the recognition of the need to defaecate may be exacerbated by other physical problems. An old person with a disabling illness may find it hard to get to the lavatory, and so may try to suppress the call to stool. Likewise haemorrhoids or anal fissures may cause pain on straining, and thus conscious or subconscious avoidance of defaecation. Dementia may render the person unable to find a lavatory, and loss of short-term memory may mean that even if the call to stool is recognized, it may be forgotten. Hurst (1919) showed that repeatedly ignoring the call to stool led to an adaptation of the sensory mechanism so that the arrival of more faeces failed to produce an adequate call to stool. The faeces may even be propelled by reverse peristalsis into more proximal parts of the colon (Avery Jones, 1972).

Dietary Changes with Age

Recent attention in the medical and lay media has focused on the increasing refinement of the diet in developed countries. The low fibre intake characteristic of such diets has been blamed for many of the diseases more common in industrialized countries, such as haemorrhoids, appendicitis, and even heart disease and cancer. On the whole, such statements are based on epidemiological evidence, but there is no doubt that a diet low in fibre can cause constipation.

Social and Economic Factors

The diet of the elderly in general reflects that of the society in which they live. Although intake falls slightly with age, probably due to decreased energy expenditure, it has been shown (Stanton and Exton-Smith, 1970) that substantial falls occur only in those whose health has deteriorated. However, many factors may contribute to the old person's food choice, and this may affect their fibre intake.

Ignorance of food values is a real problem. Brought up in times of financial hardship, and experiencing long periods of food rationing, older people have often formed poor nutritional habits which are hard to break (Thomas, 1982). However, this can be altered by education; contrary to popular belief, elderly people are willing to change their diet, especially if they receive information about the health benefits of such changes (Bilderbeck et al., 1981).

A well-balanced diet can prove expensive, and even well-motivated people may allow their diet to suffer because of economic difficulties. Income is almost always reduced on reaching retirement age, and it is reported that 23 per cent of retirement pensioners are at the officially defined subsistence level, with thousands more below it (Jordan, 1978). Reduced income can lead to a heavier reliance on Social Services (Exton-Smith and Stanton, 1965), and subsequent conflict as to how to spend what money is available; often an elderly person feels the need to choose between better food and fuel for heating.

The effects of living alone can also influence food intake. The Stockport Survey showed that people living alone have a poorer diet than those living with others (Brockington and Lempert, 1966). Attendance at luncheon clubs has been shown to improve intake, and this is likely to be for social reasons as well as for economy or convenience. Eating is a social ritual which loses some of its meaning in isolation (Thomas, 1982), and it is not surprising that the widowed in particular show less inclination to prepare nutritious meals.

Physical and Psychological Factors

There are many physical problems which affect food choice. Poor dentition makes chewing difficult, and may cause an old person to choose only soft foods. This obviously has an effect on fibre intake. Neill (1972) and Neill and Phillips (1970) claim that appetite and overall intake are unaffected; it seems that the problem is more one of specific low intake of certain foods.

Ascorbic acid intake in particular is likely to fall when fresh fruit and vegetables can no longer be chewed (Hamdy, 1984). Thomas (1980) found that 50 per cent of the elderly psychiatric patients in one survey were receiving a pureed diet, largely due to the nursing staff's fears that they might choke. It is probable that the fibre intake of these patients was markedly reduced.

Exercise

Lack of exercise is commonly associated with constipation. As previously mentioned, post-prandial propulsive movements of the gut are effective only in active people (Holdstock *et al.*, 1970). The elderly almost universally take less exercise than their younger counterparts, and so may be at risk from this factor. In particular, the ill and institutionalized old may lead a very sedentary life. Debility for any reason is also frequently associated with constipation (Hinton, 1972), as is hospitalization (Smith, 1984) both because of the lack of exercise, and on occasion because of the difficulties of using a bedpan.

Iatrogenic Constipation

Many drugs have constipation as a side-effect. Often, it is sufficient to increase fibre intake to counteract this, but on occasion aperients may be needed. The most commonly used constipating drugs are anaesthetics and muscle relaxants, ganglion blocking agents, morphine, codeine, phenytoin, anticholinergics, monoamine oxidase inhibitors and antacids. In addition, drugs such as iron compounds, diuretics and some psychotropic drugs can cause constipation in large doses or susceptible patients.

Psychiatric Problems

Constipation is associated with many psychiatric illnesses, for instance anorexia nervosa, chronic psychoses and denial of bowel actions. The most important from the point of view of the elderly is depression, which is not uncommon in this age group. The diagnosis may not always be easy (Avery Jones, 1972), especially in those patients with agitated depression.

Monitoring Constipation

Bowel habits often prove extremely difficult to monitor. Individuals frequently have differing ideas about what constitutes 'normality' and so may report problems when in fact their bowel habit is well within normal ranges. Conversely, people may not recognize constipation if they have a daily bowel action, but that action is hard and small. Burkitt has said 'It is no good having a bowel action every day, if all those stools are a week late', and this aptly describes the situation in which many patients find themselves.

It is no easier to monitor patients' bowel habits in hospital. The advent of the nursing process and patient allocation has brought evaluation of care to the centre stage, but it can still be hard to keep a check on patients, particularly those fit enough to attend to their own toilet needs. Too often constipation goes unrecognized until impaction has occurred, occasionally leading to overflow and spurious diarrhoea. The host of other problems, such as urinary incontinence, which may be caused by faecal impaction are sufficiently important to make careful bowel monitoring a vital part of the management of in-patients.

For the majority of patients, it will be sufficient simply to record the frequency and consistency of bowel movements. A day or two with no bowel movement will do no harm, but constipation more marked than this should be noted, and corrective measures instituted. Often all that is necessary is to ensure adequate fluid and fibre, plus improvement of mobility where possible. Clearly, there will be patients who need chemical laxatives, but simple monitoring as above should establish when treatment may be withdrawn, or replaced by dietary methods.

Occasionally it is necessary to perform more sophisticated monitoring of bowel habits. This is particularly the case when it is wished to evaluate a new treatment, or when two or more treatments are to be compared. In addition, some individual patients with suspected abnormal intestinal transit times may benefit from closer monitoring. Ideally, the monitoring system used should be accurate, sensitive, have no effect upon bowel habit, and be simple and inoffensive to carry out. Many methods have been devised in an attempt to achieve this ideal.

Measuring Mean Intestinal Transit Time (MTT)

Most methods of measuring transit time involve plotting the passage of some inert marker through the gut. Frequently, this involves the ingestion of the marker, and collection or observation of subsequent stools to determine the rate of passage from mouth to anus. Many different markers have been proposed, each with their attendant advantages and disadvantages.

Dyes such as carmine and charcoal have been used as a method of identifying the start and finish of different dietary periods. These are just bright dyes which colour the stool, and simply by observation give an indication of transit time. They have the advantage that lengthy stool collections are not required, but they are now rarely used as a means of estimating MTT, as single doses of marker are felt to be inaccurate.

Many other markers require the collection of stools for analysis. Investigators have used such varied markers as copper thiocyanate (Dick, 1967) and chromium sesquioxide (Davignon, Simmonds and Ahrens, 1968). Often lengthy stool collections are required to retrieve the marker, and frequently laboratory assistance is necessary to analyse the amount present. This can make the procedure slow and expensive and clearly, in an ill population, requires a great deal of co-operation from nursing staff to ensure that stool collections are maintained. Most of the methods of estimating MTT were developed and validated with fit, able groups such as university students and staff (Cummings and Wiggins 1976; Cummings, Jenkins and Wiggins, 1976), nuns (McLean Baird *et al.*, 1977) or other healthy volunteer populations. Such groups could be expected to maintain their own collections; in an inpatient population this may not be possible, and sources of human error are immediately increased.

In addition to such chemical markers as described above, investigators have used physical markers. These have included such diverse substances as coloured glass beads (Alvarez and Friedlander, 1924), tomato, millet and grape seeds, knots of cotton and ball-bearings (Hoelzel, 1930; Burnett, 1923). Again, such markers require that the stools be collected for varying periods of time, and also that they be sieved to retrieve the markers. These methods are thus subject to the problems mentioned above in collecting stools, and additionally have the disadvantage of requiring substantial handling of the specimen.

Other methods used have involved plotting the passage along the gut of a radiotelemetering capsule (Connell and Rowlands, 1960; Holdstock *et al.*, 1970) or radioisotope capsules (Kirwan and Smith, 1974; Smith *et al.*, 1980). These are useful methods, but tend to be unsuitable for epidemiological studies (Cummings and Wiggins, 1976).

The use of radio-opaque markers is now widely accepted in the measurement of MTT. Many variations of the techniques have been used. Hinton, Lennard-Jones and Young (1969) administered 20 small radio-opaque pellets to their subjects with breakfast, and collected stools until 80 per cent of the pellets had been retrieved. They measured retrieval by X-raying stools, but noted that disappearance of markers from the gut could also be measured by abdominal radiograph.

Cummings and Wiggins (1976) describe three methods of measuring MTT. They administered five radio-opaque pellets with each meal to subjects for periods from 4–12 weeks and collected all stools for X-ray. MTT was calculated from the total marker input minus the total marker recovery. Clearly, this is an exacting technique which has high reliability but is likely to be of limited use in individual patients or large-scale studies.

In addition, they describe a technique whereby subjects received, with breakfast, 20 radio-opaque pellets for three days. Each day the pellets were of different shape, and X-ray analysis of a single stool collected on the fourth day was used to estimate transit time. This was computed using the equation:

$$ \text{MTT} = \frac{t_1 s_1 + t_2 s_2}{s_1 + s_2} $$

where t_1 and t_2 are the intervals (hours) from ingestion of the two markers present in greatest numbers to the time the stool is passed, and s_1 and s_2 are the numbers of each marker present.

Finally, they computed MTT by studying the time taken from ingestion of any single dose of 20 markers to its complete recovery in the stools (as measured by X-ray).

They concluded at the end of the study that the use of a single stool to measure MTT was justified where transit time did not exceed four days. However, they do suggest that in a constipated population with slow transit times, selection of a stool later than four days should be considered.

The use of any of these methods in an elderly, constipated population has disadvantages. Any method requiring collection of stools over a period of time is likely to be associated with low compliance because of the distasteful nature of the collection. Odour-free 'collection kits' have been developed, but even so the task is unpleasant. The problems associated with 24-hour urine collections are well-known to ward staff; trying to collect several days of stools is clearly even more difficult. Even when staff are well motivated and enthusiastic, it can be extremely hard to ensure that all staff members know that the collection is being carried out, and harder to ensure that no one forgets!

The method of Cummings and Wiggins (1976) involving collection of a single stool reduces these problems to a minimum. Yet there can still be difficulties if the population is an elderly, constipated one; in order to decide on the day to be used for collection, it is necessary to collect several day's stools, at least in some patients. Only by doing this can the most representative day for that population be assessed. Therefore, in the study described below, a new variation of the method had to be used.

The study described was a clinical trial comparing lactulose with a new product, lactitol, in the treatment of constipation in the elderly. Recent proposals by the Committee on Safety of Medicines require that, in future, all drugs likely to be used by the elderly must be tested in the elderly. Before a product licence can be issued therefore, it is vital that sufficient data on old people are available.

The high laxative usage rate mentioned earlier emphasizes the need to exercise care in the prescribing of aperients to the elderly. Davison (1981) reports a high incidence of adverse drug reactions in the elderly, due he says to polypharmacy, inappropriate prescribing and altered pharmacology of the aged. It is obvious that a safe aperient with minimal side-effects could be of benefit in the field of geriatrics.

Laxatives are commonly divided into five groups; bulk-forming drugs, stimulant laxatives, faecal softeners, osmotic laxatives and rectally administered preparations. For many preparations the exact mode of action is not understood.

Lactulose and lactitol are both osmotic laxatives. Lactulose is a semi-synthetic disaccharide which is not absorbed from the gut, and which produces an osmotic diarrhoea of low pH. It is used in the treatment of hepatic encephalopathy and as an aperient. It is presented as an elixir.

Lactitol is similar to lactulose in its mode of action, but is presented in powder form. It is less sweet than lactulose, but behaves in a similar manner. It is claimed to have the same therapeutic effects as lactulose but with fewer side-effects, both in the treatment of hepatic encephalopathy and as an aperient. This study aimed to compare the efficacy, palatability, acceptability and side-effects of lactitol with lactulose, when used as an aperient in an elderly population with chronic complaints of constipation.

Design

The study was an open comparative study in patients requiring regular treatment with either laxatives or suppositories. Subjects were aged 65 or over, of either sex. The trial ran over a period of four weeks, comprising a one-week period when no oral aperients were given, followed by a three-week trial period with the subject randomly assigned to treatment with either lactulose syrup (Duphalac) or lactitol (a white crystalline powder). The initial regime was lactulose 15 ml bd, or lactitol 10 g bd, but the dose was then individually tailored to produce one or two soft stools within 24 hours of administration. The dose schedule was reviewed twice weekly.

The study was approved by the local ethics committee and witnessed verbal consent to participate was obtained by subjects or their next-of-kin.

Exclusion Criteria

(1) All patients with an organic cause for constipation.
(2) Patients with poorly-controlled diabetes mellitus.
(3) Patients with galactosaemia.
(4) Patients with lactose or sorbitol intolerance.

Subjects

Fifty-five patients were entered into the study. Forty-two completed the four-week trial period, of which 32 had MTT measured as described below. The mean age of subjects was 81.9 (range 67–99). Mean mental test score as measured by the method of Qureshi and Hodkinson (1974) was 5.9 out of a possible maximum of ten (range 0–10). A score of seven or less is taken to indicate significant impairment. Nine patients lived at home but attended the Day Hospital at St Pancras Hospital. The remainder were inpatients at either St Pancras Hospital or Hornsey Central Hospital. Seventeen were independently mobile (with or without aids), eight needed assistance and seventeen were immobile.

To ensure that allocation to treatment groups was random, difference between means for age and mental score was assessed by Student's t-test and was not significant for either parameter. Other parameters were assessed by chi-squared. No significant differences were found in the patient characteristics of either treatment group.

Methods of Measurement

Efficacy

Relative MTT was estimated by the administration of 20 radio-opaque markers per day to all subjects throughout the trial period, in a similar manner to that of Andersson *et al.* (1985). The markers were made from radio-opaque tubing (external diameter 3.0 mm) and were enclosed in a gelatine capsule for ease of swallowing. They were administered during the morning drug round (usually about 9.00 a.m.).

By the final week, marker ingestion and excretion were assumed to have equilibrated, even in the most constipated subjects. A plain abdominal X-ray was then taken. This allowed the markers to be counted, and relative transit times to be estimated. A high number of markers indicates that transit time is slow, whilst a low number of markers indicates a rapid transit.

In addition, patients' bowel actions were recorded daily throughout the trial period. The number of patients who required enemata, either during the pretreatment phase or whilst receiving the aperient, was also recorded.

Palatability

Measuring palatability is difficult and subjective. A significant number of patients had a degree of dementia, and were thus unable to give an opinion of taste etc. Palatability for these patients was assessed by asking staff how willingly the preparation was taken in relation to other medications. Patients who were able to give an opinion were asked to rate taste as 'excellent', 'good', 'indifferent' or 'poor'.

Side-effects

Full blood count (including differential white cell count) and biochemistry screen including urea and electrolytes were carried out. Urine was analysed for pH and calcium/creatinine ratio.

Such symptoms as flatulence, cramps, etc. are more nebulous and difficult to review. Informal, semi-structured interviews with staff and patients, carried out frequently (twice per week), proved the most effective method of eliciting the information desired.

Results

Withdrawals

There were thirteen withdrawals, none of which was due to either treatment. Four patients were discharged, with follow-up at home judged to be impracticable. Two patients were deemed unfit to start the treatment phase of the trial, one because of impaction and one because of abnormal biochemistry results. Two others developed acute illnesses during the trial necessitating their withdrawal (one had CVA and was unconscious, one was transferred to another hospital following a fall). Three patients died after recruitment; none had started the treatment phase and none of the deaths were expected. One patient withdrew her consent, and one was withdrawn after the ward staff stopped both the treatment and the capsules.

Mean Intestinal Transit Time

The pellet counts for each treatment phase are as shown in Table 1.

Table 1 Pellet count

	Mean	SD
Lactitol ($n = 19$)	103	53
Lactulose ($n = 13$)	99	75

The difference between the means was calculated using t-test modification for small sample sizes and was not significant.

The distribution of the pellet counts within the treatment groups was compared using Wilcoxon's rank sum test, as the count was slightly skewed (median 95, range 2–238). The difference in distribution was not significant ($p < 0.1$)

The results were analysed using a multiple regression technique. The pellet count was taken as the dependent variable, and the age, sex, standardized aperient dose, and drug administered were used as independent variables. The standard dose of the drug was calculated by dividing the subject's cumulative dose by the mean cumulative dose (mean cumulative dose = 450 for patients taking lactitol, and = 629 for patients taking lactulose). This allows direct comparison between the two drugs as it eliminates the differences in strength and presentation of the medication.

No differences were found at 5 per cent significance level for any single variable, or for any combinations of variables. There was a trend toward a higher pellet count with increasing age which was significant only at the 6 per cent level. On further analysis corrected to take into account the skew, this was confirmed as not significant. This agrees with the studies of Connell *et al.* (1965) and Milne and Williamson (1972), who showed no age changes in gut transit time.

The difference between the mean number of bowel movements per week (see Table 2) was assessed by Student's t-test, examining the difference between the treatment groups for each observation phase, and for the difference between the pretreatment and treatment phases. The number of patients requiring enemata was similarly assessed using chi-square. No difference between the two treatment groups was found, but both significantly increased the mean number of bowel movements per patient week, and reduced the number of enemata required.

Table 2   Bowel movements

	Pre-treatment (1 week)		Treatment phase (3 weeks)	
	Mean no. BMs/week	No. patients requiring enemas	Mean no. BMs/week	No. patients requiring enemas
Lactitol	2.8	14	4.5	9
Lactulose	3.0	9	4.5	4

Palatability

The majority of patients in both groups reported that the taste was 'indifferent'. Taste was rated as 'poor' by one subject taking lactitol, and three taking lactulose. It was rated as 'good' or 'excellent' by six subjects taking lactitol, and one taking lactulose. This was analysed by chi-squared and is not significant.

However, some staff did report that sprinkling lactitol onto food made it easier to administer to some patients, and it was the subjective opinion of the researcher that lactitol was preferred. The large proportion of patients reporting the taste as 'indifferent' may have masked any minor preference.

Side-effects

The number of patients reporting side-effects was small. Therefore, analysis of each side-effect was carried out using *any* report of that problem, even if this was mild, or reported only once during the trial period (see Table 3).

Table 3   Side-effects

Side-effect	Number of patients reporting Lactitol	Lactulose	Yates's chi-square	Significance
Meteorism	4	5	0.24	NS
Flatulence	9	9	0.25	NS
Abdominal cramp	11	7	0.02	NS
Diarrhoea	6	5	0.02	NS

Meteorism refers to an urgency in the desire to defaecate, coupled with rapid defaecation, but without looseness of stools.

Nausea was not a problem for any patient taking lactulose, but was reported by three patients taking lactitol. Because of the small numbers, Fisher's exact test was used to analyse this response. No statistically significant difference was found.

Only one patient (taking lactulose) reported pruritis ani. This patient had urinary incontinence and an associated dermatitis involving the perineum, and it was assumed that this was the real cause of the pruritis.

Laboratory Analyses

It must be remembered that the population studied was made up largely of in-patients, and that all participants were receiving hospital treatment. It is therefore to be expected that a high proportion of patients would show biochemical/haematological abnormalities. During the study, any abnormal results were brought to the attention of the patient's physician, and the possibility of any connection with the trial was discussed.

Only one patient was denied entry to the trial because of biochemical/haematological abnormalities. Abnormalities were detected on initial screening for many other patients, but they were not considered to be such as to warrant their non-inclusion.

Thirty-one patients showed changes in laboratory results over the period of the trial, with seventeen showing a return to normal, and fourteen changing from normal to abnormal. The difference between the two is not significant. There was no detectable pattern in these changes, and none appeared clinically important.

Discussion of Trial Results

No difference in efficacy was found between the two treatment groups. This is to be expected as both are claimed to have the same mode of action. From the results obtained, it would seem that lactitol and lactulose are comparable in their efficacy when used in the treatment of chronic constipation in the elderly.

No differences were found between the treatments in terms of side-effects, both with regard to laboratory parameters and subjective side-effects. The results indicate that the two drugs are comparable in this respect.

No significant difference was found between the two drugs in terms of taste. However, there was an apparent preference for lactitol which did not reach significant levels. It is possible that the method of questioning masked any true preference as so many subjects reported the taste as 'indifferent'. A further study examining taste preference could be usefully carried out to establish the likelihood of this trend reaching significant levels.

In conclusion, it would appear that lactitol is as effective, as well tolerated and possibly more palatable than lactulose, when used in the treatment of constipation in elderly people.

Discussion of Method of Measuring MTT

This trial can be criticized on several methodological points. It would have been of more value to have used a crossover design so that all patients had a period of treatment with both drugs. In addition, to have carried out measurements of MTT on patients both before and after treatment would have made more information available on individuals. This was not done because of constraints of time, plus the fact that within the remit of the trial, the most important aspect was the *group* response, i.e. whether the group of patients on lactitol had a different MTT from the group on lactulose.

Accepting these limitations, the trial does give some interesting information on the feasibility of using this method to estimate relative MTT. Despite the exacting nature of the method, 32 of the 42 completed patients had MTT estimated (76 per cent). The subjects who did not have MTT measured either:

(a) Forgot (or refused) to take the capsules.
(b) Refused to have the X-ray.
(c) Were unable (because of frailty) to have the X-ray.

None failed to have MTT successfully estimated because of error on the part of either the investigator or the nursing staff. It is possible that an even higher number might have had MTT estimated if it had been possible to monitor more closely those patients who lived at home, as the majority of those who forgot their capsules were not inpatients. In addition, to have arranged to have the markers in two smaller gelatine capsules rather than the one used might also have helped. The capsule used was only the size of a 500 mg antibiotic capsule, but even so one or two patients did refuse it on the grounds of size alone.

As has been noted, this method was used to estimate group MTT. However, there would seem to be no reason why it could not be used to examine individual bowel habits. Repeat estimates could easily be made to compare MTT on different regimes of care within the same subject. A study to examine the sensitivity to change of this method could perhaps usefully be carried out. In this study, the absolute number of pellets on the X-ray was all that was recorded, but it would be a simple matter to convert this to an estimate of MTT in days.

The main advantage of this technique is that it requires so little effort from either subject or carers, as virtually the only thing which has to be remembered is to take the marker. In hospital this is easily dealt with by including the capsule in the routine drug round and even when subjects are at home, the majority can comply with support from the investigator. No stool collections are required, so the method is also aesthetically more acceptable to all involved. In addition, no specialized equipment is needed to perform the measurement; access to X-ray equipment can be arranged for most subjects wherever they are, even though access to radiotelemetering facilities, etc., might be impossible.

Such considerations are especially important when dealing with an elderly population. The concern is often expressed that the old should 'not be bothered with all these complicated tests'. To measure MTT by one of the more usual methods would only rarely be justifiable in an elderly population; the method outlined above could, however, be used on a much wider group of subjects.

References

Alvarez, W. C., and Friedlander, B. L. (1924). The rate of progress of food residues through the bowel. *J. Am. Med. Assoc*, **83**, 576–580.

Andersson, H., Ryba, W., Stener, I. and Stenquist, B. (1985). Colonic transit after fibre supplementation in patients with haemorrhoids. *Hum. Nutr. Appl. Nutr.*, **39A**, 101–107.

Avery-Jones, F. (1972). Management of constipation in adults, in Avery-Jones,

F. and Godding, E. W., *Management of Constipation*. Blackwell Scientific Publications, Oxford.

Bhanthumnavin, K. and Schuster, M. (1977). Aging and gastrointestinal function, in Finch, C. E. and Hayflick, L., *Handbook of the Biology of Aging*. Van Nostrand Reinhold Company, New York.

Bilderbeck, N., Holdsworth, M. D., Purves, R. and Davies, L. (1981). Changing food habits among 100 elderly men and women in the United Kingdom. *J. Hum. Nutr.*, **35** (6), 448–455.

Brockington, F. and Lempert, S. M. (1966). Stockport Survey. The Social Needs of the over 80s. Manchester: University Press.

Burnett, F. L. (1923). The intestinal rate and the form of the faeces. *Am. J. Roent*, **10**, 599–604.

Connell, A., Hilton, C., Irvine, G., Lennard-Jones, J. and Misciewicz, J. (1965). Variation of bowel habit in two population samples. *Brit. Med. J.*, **ii**, 1095.

Connell, A. M. and Rowlands, E. N. (1960). Wireless telemetering from the digestive tract. *Gut*, **1**, 266–272.

Connell, A. M. (1972). Physiology of the colon, in Avery-Jones, F. and Godding, E. W., *Management of Constipation*. Blackwell Scientific Publications, Oxford.

Cummings, J. H., Jenkins, D. J. A. and Wiggins, H. S. (1976). Measurement of the mean transit time of dietary residue through the human gut. *Gut*, **17**, 216–218.

Cummings, J. H. and Wiggins, H. S. (1976). Transit through the gut measured by analysis of a single stool. *Gut*, **17**, 219–223.

Davignon, J., Simmonds, W. J. and Ahrens, E. H. jr (1968). Usefulness of chromic oxide as an internal standard for balance studies in formula-fed patients and for assessment of colonic function. *J. Clin. Invest.*, **47**, 127–138.

Davison, W., (1981). Prescribing for the elderly. *Practitioner*, **225**, 1727–1735.

Dick, M. (1967). Use of barium sulphate as a continuous marker for faeces. *J. Clin. Path.*, **20**, 216–218.

Dick, M. (1969). Use of cuprous thiocyanate as a short-term continuous marker for faeces. *Gut*, **10**, 408–412.

Exton-Smith, A. N. (1972). Constipation in geriatrics, E. W. in Avery-Jones, F. and Godding, E. W. *Management of Constipation*. Blackwell Scientific Publications, Oxford.

Frenckner, B. and Ihre, T. (1976). Influence of the autonomic nerves on the internal anal sphincter in man. *Gut*, 17, 306–312.

Hamdy, R. C. (1984). *Geriatric Medicine — a Problem-orientated Approach*. Baillière Tindall, Eastbourne.

Hinton, J. M. Lennard-Jones, J. E. and Young, A. C. (1969). A new method for studying gut transit times using radioopaque markers. *Gut*, **10**, 842–847.

Hinton, J. M. (1972). Diagnosis, in Avery-Jones, F. and Godding, E. W. (Eds), *Management of Constipation*. Blackwell Scientific Publications, Oxford.

Hoelzel, F. (1930). The rate of passage of inert materials through the digestive tract. *Am. J. Physiol*, **92**, 466–497.

Holdstock, D. J., Misciewicz, J. J., Smith, T. and Rowlands, E. N. (1970). Propulsion (mass movements) in the human colon and its relationship to meals and somatic activity. *Gut*, **11**, 91–99.

Hurst, A. F. (1919). *Constipation and Allied Disorders (2nd Edn)*. Oxford University Press, London.

Jordan, D. (1978). Poverty and the elderly, in Carver, and Liddiard (Eds), *An Ageing Population*. Open University Press, Kent.

Kirwan, W. D. and Smith, A. N. (1974). Gastrointestinal transit estimated by an isotope capsule. *Scand. J. Gastroenterol*, **9**, 763–769.

McLean, Baird I., Walters, R. L., Davies, P. S., Hill, M. J., Drasar, B. S. and Southgate, D.A.T. (1977). The effects of two dietary supplements on gastrointestinal transit, stool weight and frequency, and bacterial flors, and bile acids in normal subjects. *Metabolism*, **26** (2), 117–127.

Mars, G. and Buogo, A. (1967). Considerazioni sui diverticoli del colon nell eta avanzata. *G. Geront.*, **15**, 1243–1266.

Milne, J. S. and Williamson, J. (1972). Bowel habit in older people. *Geront clin*, **14**, 56–60.

Neill, D. J. (1972). Masticatory studies, in *A Nutritional Survey of the Elderly — Report of the Panel on Nutrition of the Elderly*. DHSS, London, HMSO.

Neill, D. J. and Philips, H. I. (1970). The masticatory performance, dental state and dietary intake of a group of army pensioners. *Brit. Dent. J.*, **128**, 581–585.

Newman, H. F. and Freeman, J. (1974). Physiologic factors affecting defecatory sensation. *J. Am. Geriat. Soc.*, **22**, 553–554.

Parks, J. W. (1943). Bowel habit and investigation based on the examination of 1115 male adults. MD Thesis (Cambridge).

Qureshi, K. N. and Hodkinson, H. M. (1974). Evaluation of a ten question mental test in the institutionalized elderly. *Age and Ageing*, **3**, 152–157.

Smith, R., Rowe, M., Smith, A., Eastwood, M., Drummond, E. and Brydon, W. G. (1980). A study of bulking agents in elderly patients. *Age and Ageing*, **9**, 267–271.

Smith, R. (1984). Preventing and treating constipation. *Geriatrics for GPs*, **14** (11), 32–35.

Stanton, B. and Exton-Smith, A. N. (1970). *A Longitudinal Study of the Dietary of Elderly Women*. KEHFL, London.

Thomas, S. (1982). The elderly — a forgotten nutrition problem? *Getting the Most Out of Food*. Van den Burghs and Jurgens Nutrition Education Service.

Thomas, S. J. (1980). A study of the nutritional status of longstay patients in Springfield Hospital. Unpublished, copies available from Geriatric Teaching and Research Unit, St George's Hospital, Blackshaw Rd, London SW17.

Warren, R. (1978). Age changes in intestinal mucosa. *Lancet*, **II**, 849.

Yamagata, A. (1965). Histopathological studies of the colon in relation to age. *Jap. J. Gastroent.*, **62**, 229–235.

Research in the Nursing Care of Elderly People
Edited by P. Fielding
Published (1987) by John Wiley & Sons Ltd
© Crown Copyright Reserved 1986

CHAPTER 3

Developments in the Provision and Evaluation of Long-term Care for Dependent Old People

JOHN BOND and SENGA BOND

Introduction

Since the inception of the National Health Service (NHS) in 1948 there has been an increase in the number and proportion of the population reaching retirement age (65 for men and 60 for women). In 1951 10.9 per cent of the population of the United Kingdom were aged 65 or over and 0.4 per cent were aged 85 or over. In 1981 these proportions had increased to 15.1 per cent and 1.1 per cent respectively. However, current demographic predictions suggest that although the proportion of the population aged 65 or over will remain fairly constant the proportion aged 85 or over will continue to rise in the next thirty years to about 2.1 per cent of the population. With a stable population these increases in proportion reflect the increase in the absolute numbers of elderly people, particularly those aged 85 or over who will increase in number from about 200 000 in 1951 to an estimated 1.2 million in 2011 (Office of Population, Censuses and Surveys, 1986). It has been estimated that of those aged 85 or over one in five might suffer from moderate or severe dementia (Report of the Royal College of Physicians, 1981) and three in five a limiting long-standing illness (Office of Population, Censuses and Surveys, 1982).

Since 1948 the long-term care of elderly people has been provided by the families of elderly people and by the private, statutory and voluntary sectors. Families continue to provide the majority of care (Wicks and Rossiter, 1982; Parker, 1985) but where family care has not been available dependent elderly people have always been cared for in

47

a variety of institutions (Thomson, 1983). Institutional care for elderly people currently includes local authority and voluntary residential homes, private rest homes, NHS and private nursing homes, and acute, geriatric and psychiatric NHS hospital wards.

Since 1948 there has been a substantial amount of research of variable quality focusing on the long-term care of elderly people. Reviews of this literature suggest that there is considerable consensus about a number of features of that care:

1   There is great variability in both the quantity and quality of services for elderly people across the country. In particular, the statutory authorities operate different policies in the organization of services, leading to a different kind of service being offered (Davies et al., 1971; Williamson, 1979; Wade, Sawyer and Bell, 1983; Brocklehurst and Andrews, 1985).

2   In NHS hospitals many general medical beds are perceived as 'blocked' by elderly people requiring long-term residential accommodation or are 'misplaced' in the care system; implying that there is a scarcity of this facility (Kidd, 1962; McKeown and Cross, 1969; Langley and Simpson, 1970; Carstairs and Morison, 1971; Evans, Hodkinson and Mezey, 1971; Gelding and Newell, 1972; Hodkinson, Evans and Mezey, 1972; McKechnie, 1972; Brocklehurst, 1975; Copeland et al., 1975; McArdle, Wylie and Alexander, 1975; Rubin and Davies, 1975; Plank, 1977; Brocklehurst et al., 1978; Roe and Guillem, 1978; Currie, Smith and Williamson, 1979; Covell and Angus, 1980; Coid and Crome, 1986).

3   As a result of this perceived scarcity admission to NHS hospital beds and local authority residential care appears to be mainly 'crisis based' (Barnes, 1980) and for 'social reasons' (Townsend, 1965; Isaacs, Livingstone and Neville, 1972; Berkeley, 1976; Farrow, Rablen and Silver, 1976; Bond and Carstairs, 1982; Graham and Livesley, 1983; Booth, 1985).

4   There is considerable overlap between the characteristics of elderly people living in private households, sheltered housing, local authority residential homes, private rest homes, private nursing homes and different types of NHS hospitals (Townsend, 1962; Townsend and Wedderburn, 1965; McKeown and Cross, 1969; Carstairs and Morison, 1971; Isaacs and Neville, 1975; Plank, 1977; Wilkin, Mashiah and Jolley, 1978; Gilleard, 1980; Bond and Carstairs, 1982). In addition, it has been confirmed that for every severely physically incapacitated elderly person living in an institution there

are four living in private households either alone or with other elderly people or in other types of households (Townsend and Wedderburn, 1965; Bond and Carstairs, 1982). However, for every one elderly person with a diagnosis of moderate or severe dementia or confusion living at home there are three in institutions (Bond, 1987).

5   There would appear to be considerable numbers of elderly people living in private households whom professionals deem to be in need of services, but for whom no service is provided (Townsend, 1957; Townsend, 1962; Williamson et al., 1964; Townsend and Wedderburn, 1965; Harris, 1968; Hunt, 1970; Andrews, Cowan and Anderson, 1971; Cartwright, Hockey and Anderson, 1973; Townsend, 1973; Powell and Crombie, 1974; Marks, 1975; Gardiner, 1975; Gruer, 1975; Isaacs and Neville, 1975; Foster, Kay and Bergmann, 1976; Bond and Carstairs, 1982).

6   Finally, there is considerable evidence of strain on carers of elderly people living in private households which has led to crisis admissions and detrimental effects on carers (Hoenig and Hamilton, 1966; Grad and Sainsbury, 1968; Droller, 1969; Isaacs, 1971; Cresswell and Pasker, 1972; Isaacs, Livingstone and Neville, 1972; Cartwright, Hockey and Anderson, 1973; Sanford, 1975; Bergmann et al., 1978; Equal Opportunities Commission, 1980; Brocklehurst et al., 1981; Charlesworth, Wilkin and Durie, 1984; Jones & Vetter, 1984).

In this chapter we will the use term *long-term institutional care* to refer to the type of care provided by private rest homes, local authority and voluntary residential homes, private and NHS nursing homes and long-stay geriatric and psychogeriatric hospital wards. When referring to elderly people, we will restrict the term patient to people in hospital and use the term resident for people who are in institutional care. The chapter briefly reviews developments in long-term institutional care for elderly people before exploring a framework for its evaluation.

Developments in Long-term Institutional Care

Although there has been continuing promotion of community care for elderly people (DHSS, 1982), the reality is that community care means care by the family and care by the family means care by women (Finch and Groves, 1983). However, the absence of family support has been shown to be a major reason for admission to an institution (Townsend, 1965; Isaacs, Livingstone and Neville, 1972; Bond and Carstairs, 1982) and there is likely always to be a demand for some kind of institutional care. Developments in the provision of long-term institutional care must also be set against the backcloth of a dramatic increase in the numbers of people aged 85 or over.

The United Kingdom is one of the few industrialized countries which provides a specialist service for the medical care of elderly people (Brocklehurst, 1975). However, throughout the UK this service takes on a variety of forms. Williamson (1979) has characterized three stages in the development of geriatric medicine. The first stage, exemplified by the pioneers of geriatric medicine (Warren, 1949; Adams, 1952), focused on the institutional care of chronically ill people and the development of the distinction between acute, rehabilitative and long-stay care (Adams, 1964). The second stage represented the movement towards the community and was characterized by the introduction of domiciliary visits and closer links with general practitioners, and the development of other community services. The third stage recognized the preventative aspects of geriatric medicine with increased emphasis on the role of primary health care services (Andrews, Cowan and Anderson, 1971). Thus the work of Departments of Geriatric Medicine has steadily expanded and currently comprises a wide range of activities, but in general, all departments set out to provide a service for a defined population and provide a comprehensive range of facilities. However, there is great variation in the type of patient admitted, from acutely ill patients to much more chronically ill patients. A fourth stage in the development of geriatric medicine focuses on changes toward the elimination of long-stay beds and the discharging of all long-stay patients from hospital.

The development of geriatric medicine has strongly influenced the organization of the nursing of elderly people. Evers (1981) and Kitson (1984) among others have stressed that nursing has failed to define its caring role despite the pioneering work of Norton, McLaren and Exton-Smith (1962). Evers attributes this to the prevailing dominant and oppressive medical model while Kitson regards the cause as the absence of any theoretical model underpinning care. Wells (1980) also notes that the absence of specific knowledge, which will inform nurses why they do what they do, is due to a failure of nursing to define clearly its area of practice and functions. The way patient care is medically organized has been attributed by Brocklehurst (1978) and Hodkinson (1981) to the convenience and morale of nurses, rather than to patient welfare. How the organization of in-patient geriatric services influences the care of long-stay patients has not been investigated but the acute medical model which stresses recovery and discharge prevails. That there is a role for nurses in the long-term care of elderly people has rarely been questioned. Yet Miller and Gwynne (1972) and Halliburton and Wright (1974) have suggested that nurses are not the most appropriate providers of care in long-term settings. This may explain why heads of local authority residential homes are unlikely to have a nursing background.

Under the terms of the 1948 National Assistance Act local authorities are required to provide residential care for dependent people. Since 1948 there has been a change in the condition of old people's homes. More residential homes are now purpose built for the care of disabled people. With the increasing numbers of mentally impaired elderly people entering residential homes some authorities have developed separate facilities for the elderly mentally infirm; in the form of either separate units within existing homes or separate homes.

Of increasing importance in recent years has been the development of a flourishing private sector. The availability of alternative residential care for elderly people also has a reciprocal effect on the demand for local authority residential homes and the work of departments of geriatric medicine.

In some areas, particularly in the coastal retirement areas there has always been a flourishing private sector. Until recently almost all residents of private rest and nursing homes were self-financed. Following the 1979 supplementary benefit regulations, residents in private nursing and rest homes became eligible for supplementary benefit. Until 1983 there were varying interpretations of the Act so that local DHSS officers set different levels of benefit. Variations in the provision of private homes reflected differences in benefit payments. Health and local authorities also responded in different ways to the availability of private homes and thus in some areas there has been more encouragement to develop private residential facilities for elderly people.

These developments in the provision of long-term institutional care appear to be leading towards a major change in the type of institutional care provided. As geriatric medicine increasingly focuses on acute care and rehabilitation there is pressure to remove all long-stay beds from geriatric hospitals and provide nursing-home care for elderly people. Since 1979 the majority of nursing homes have been developed by the private sector and the majority of this provision has been provided by small businesses rather than the larger health care organizations although these are increasingly likely to develop nursing home type facilities while the political climate continues to support the private sector. Within the NHS the DHSS has promoted the concept of NHS nursing homes (DHSS, 1983) and these are being established in a number of health authorities. However, away from the traditional retirement areas long-term nursing care is provided predominantly in geriatric hospitals.

Characteristics of Residents in Long-term Care Institutions

Since Townsend undertook his seminal studies of institutional life in old people's homes and hospitals (Townsend, 1962; Townsend and Wedderburn, 1965; Townsend, 1973) there have been a large number of published studies which have described the characteristics of elderly people in institutions (McKeown and Cross, 1969; Carstairs and Morison, 1971; Isaacs, Livingstone and Neville, 1972; Gruer, 1975; Isaacs and Neville, 1975; Rainey, Russel and Silver, 1975; Wilkin, Mashiah and Jolley, 1978; Alexander and Eldon, 1979; Clarke et al., 1979; Dodd, Holden and Reed, 1979; Gilleard, Pattie and Dearman, 1980; Donaldson, Clayton and Clarke, 1980; Masterton, Holloway and Timbury, 1981; Twining and Allen, 1981; Bond and Carstairs, 1982; Charlesworth and Wilkin, 1982; McLauchlan and Wilkin, 1982; Wade, Sawyer and Bell, 1983; Mann, Graham and Ashby, 1984; Booth, 1985; Miller, 1985; Wright, 1985; Primrose and Capewell, 1986; Atkinson et al, 1986). While each of these studies has collected data about the behavioural characteristics of elderly patients and residents, few have used comparable methods of assessment. Some studies have focused on a particular type of institution while others have included a variety of types. The number of subjects assessed varies markedly between studies.

Although there have been a number of changes in policy since the establishment of the NHS it is remarkable that there has been little change in the proportion of people aged 65 or over living in institutions: overall, about 5 per cent. The recent expansion in the provision of private rest and nursing homes may change this stable pattern.

How have the statutory services coped with the increase in the numbers of people aged 85 or over between 1951 and 1981? Part of the explanation may be found in an expansion in community-based services, an increase in family care and the effectiveness of geriatric medicine in rehabilitating patients for discharge back into the community. Much of the increase in physical and mental incapacity resulting from demographic changes has been absorbed by institutional care. In particular, residential homes now care for a higher proportion of physically and mentally incapacitated residents (Dodd, Holden and Reed, 1979; Gilleard, Pattie and Dearman 1980; Bebbington and Tong, 1983; Booth, 1985) and there is evidence that this proportion has now stabilized (Charlesworth and Wilkin, 1982; Booth *et al.*, 1983).

Characteristics of Institutions

It has been recognized for a number of years that many long-term care institutions whatever their clientele, exhibit the characteristics of what Goffman (1961) has termed the total institution. The essential feature of the total institution, which distinguishes it from other forms of organization is that, unlike life outside, there is no separation between the three central spheres of life: work, leisure and the family. All aspects of life are conducted within the boundaries of the institution and under the control of a single authority. Each phase of daily activities is shared with a large number of other people, all of whom are treated alike and are required to do the same things together. These activities normally follow a strict routine imposed from above by a system of explicit formal rulings and a body of officials. The routine of daily activities comprises a single rational plan which has been designed to fulfil the official aims of the institution.

Detailed British studies of residential homes for elderly people (Townsend, 1962), of residential homes for the physically disabled and young chronic sick people (Miller and Gwynne, 1972), and of long-stay geriatric hospital wards (Baker, 1978; Evers, 1981) exemplify Goffman's model, although these studies also show that the concept is not relevant to all long-term institutions. As a result of these and other studies there have been various efforts to overcome the effects of institutionalization through the process of normalization: the principle that people living in institutions should be able to follow a life-style similar to the patterns they would experience living in private households (Wolfensberger, 1972).

Framework of Evaluation

Illsley (1980) has indicated the breadth of meaning given to the term evaluation and the consequent range of methods used in evaluation research. First, is the experimental study in which randomization of subjects to alternative modes of care is the essential feature. Second, is the quasi-experimental study in which a new mode of care is compared with existing modes but without the randomization of subjects. Third, is the descriptive study in which existing modes of care are described.

The essential feature of the experimental design is the random allocation of subjects to alternative modes of care. Comparison of the outcomes of the alternative modes is undertaken to inform us of the relative effectiveness of the two modes of care. However, sole reliance on outcome measures involves the practical difficulty of determining the value of various outcomes and the difficulty of knowing what features of care affect outcomes. Thus while outcome measures are a necessary component of experimental and quasi-experimental designs, they are in themselves insufficient to provide an explanation of what was influential in creating such outcomes and any differences between them.

An encompassing approach to evaluation of care is provided by Donabedian (1980) in a medical context. Donabedian's thrust is the definition of quality of medical care and approaches to assessing it. He argues that 'the most direct route to an assessment of the quality of care is an examination of that care' (1980, p. 81). This involves those activities that go on between those who provide care and the recipients and are termed the 'process of care'. Two less direct approaches to assessing quality are also available. The first is to consider the 'structure' of care, that is the relatively stable characteristics of those who provide care, the resources they have at their disposal, the physical and organizational settings in which care is provided, indeed all of those factors of production of care as well as the ways in which the financing and delivery of health services are organized, both formally and informally. Structure thus influences the kind of care that is provided by increasing or decreasing the probability of good performance.

The second indirect way to assess quality of care is to consider outcomes. Outcomes include changes in patients' current and future health status attributable to antecedent health care. These may include social, psychological, physical and physiological functioning as well as attitudes including satisfaction as components of current or as contributions to future health. Outcomes can be used as indicators of quality only in so far as the structure and process of care actually affects them. Donabedian's premise is that there is a fundamental functional relationship between the three elements, expressed as:

$$\text{Structure} \rightarrow \text{Process} \rightarrow \text{Outcome}$$

'This means that structural characteristics of the settings in which care takes place have a propensity to influence the process of care so that its quality is diminished or enhanced. Similariy, changes in the process of care, including variations in its quality, will influence the effect of care on health status, broadly defined' (Donabedian, 1980, p. 84).

From the perspective of social welfare rather than medicine, Davies and Knapp (1981) draw attention to the fundamental difference between quality of care and quality of life. This leads them to develop a model for the evaluation of institutional care, specifically old people's homes, which is explicitly based on production relations. Following this analysis quality of life and all the other benefits derived from the provision of residential care are termed 'outputs' and their determinants, that is all of the resources and non-resource contributions to residential care are termed 'inputs'. Their model can be expressed as:

$$\text{Inputs} \rightarrow \frac{\text{Intermediate}}{\text{outputs}} \rightarrow \frac{\text{Final}}{\text{outputs}}$$

They attempt to elucidate the complex production relations which exist between inputs and outputs in old peoples' homes as a means of directing research which will take account of this complexity while adhering to the central feature of the theory of production of welfare, that is the idea of fit between residents, who differ greatly in their needs, and environment. Social environment and residents' characteristics must not be viewed apart from one another.

The different terminology and emphases employed by Donabedian (1980) and by Davies and Knapp (1981) are essentially those which arise from differences in discipline and perspective. The generality of Donabedian's model and its stress on the different contributions of structure, process and outcome to evaluation of care together with the specificity of the theoretical model constructed by Davies and Knapp, emphasizing the interactive and reflexive nature of the social environment of old peoples' homes, have influenced greatly the development of our thinking.

While there is a need for research which will take account of these various features, often disciplinary and ideological differences and strong adherence to a particular methodological stance inhibit such developments. This is not to underestimate the practical difficulties which arise from variations within and between institutions and institutional regimes, differences between clientele, and differential interaction effects between the type of care delivered and recipients of care. Even if the purposes and objectives of such care can be agreed there remain problems of definition and measurement. In addition, there are practical problems of control over at least some sources of variation and the expense which research of an experimental or longitudinal nature in multiple sites entails. Worthwhile research to evaluate long-term institutional care must feature agreed outcomes of care, the means of describing the process of care and its structure, methods which permit the attribution of outcomes to antecedents, and techniques which adequately assess relevant variables. This will result in studies which include both descriptive and explanatory methods. Given these stringent, demanding and expensive requirements it is not surprising that such studies as do exist tend to be small scale, narrowly focused, and are often uncontrolled.

The proposed model shown in Figure 1 was developed for a study to evaluate experimental NHS nursing homes (Bond, 1984). However, the approach discussed here has general relevance for the evaluation of other types of long-term institutional care. In reviewing this model we begin at its end by discussing final outcomes, before reviewing in turn intermediate outcomes, process and lastly structure.

Measuring Final Outcomes

The definition of appropriate outcome measures represents the first challenge to evaluative research. What constitutes appropriate outcomes for long-term health care will depend on perspective and values. As Lemke and Moos (1986) write 'Society will continue to debate the relative values of survival, satisfaction, intact functioning, and environmental challenge in old age' (p. 275). Not only is there disagreement about the relative importance of different outcomes but appropriate outcomes are likely to vary according to different perspectives and policy objectives. Outcome measures should cover the range of care objectives and measure individual well-being on each of the dimensions relating to care objectives, using measures which are scalable, sensitive, manageable, valid and reliable. In medical research survival has been used as the predominant outcome in judging the effectiveness of a given treatment or intervention whereas personal well-being has been a feature of the social welfare model. However the importance of personal well-being is increasingly recognized by physicians responsible for long-term care and the idea of autonomy has been proposed by Evans (1984) as the global aim of all services. Recently economists have brought these two concepts together in order to estimate a measure based on quality adjusted life years (Williams, 1985; Torrance, 1986).

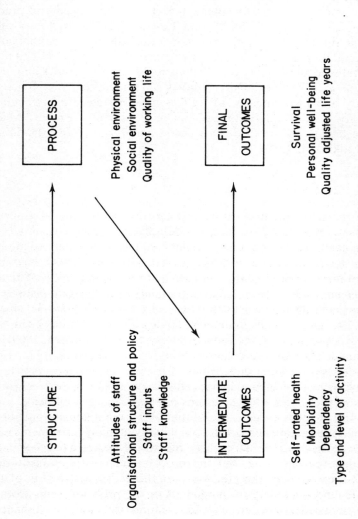

Figure 1 An evaluative model for long-term care

Survival

Differential survival rates which exist within and between types of institutions will reflect among other things the age, level of functional incapacity, morbidity and mental state of elderly people at the time of admission. Survival has been shown to be strongly associated with mental impairment (Goldfarb, 1969; Whitehead and Hunt, 1982) and has therefore been used by Christie (1982) and Blessed and Wilson (1982) among others to evaluate the changes in psychiatric practice over a 25-year period. Smith and Lowther (1976) used survival to estimate the extent of misplacement in local authority residential homes and found that mortality was greater than expected. Booth (1985) found no difference in mortality rates between old people's homes employing different care regimes. Other studies have identified that functional capacity and incontinence, as well as mental state are predictors of mortality among long-term patients and residents (Brauer, Mackeprange and Bentzon, 1978; Donaldson and Jagger, 1983; Hodkinson and Hodkinson, 1980).

Personal Well-being

Given the self-contained nature of long-stay institutions all aspects of a residents well-being are likely to be influenced by the quality of life experienced in the institution. Attempts to measure quality of life have usually focused on measures of personal satisfaction which have been devised in the United States and modified for use in the UK. The most reliable and most widely used instruments are: the Life Satisfaction Rating (Neugarten, Havighurst and Tobin, 1961); the Life Satisfaction Index (Neugarten, Havighurst and Tobin, 1961) which has been anglicized by Luker (1979); the Affect Balance Scale (Bradburn, 1969); and the Philadelphia Geriatric Centre Morale Scale (Lawton, 1972; 1975), which focuses on three dimensions of morale: depression, anxiety and negative aspects of ageing. Davies and Knapp (1981) provide a valuable review of these and other measures of psychological well-being.

Quality of life is elusive and Booth (1985) comments not only on the cultural unsuitability and construct invalidity of many instruments which purport to measure life satisfaction, morale, self-esteem or other indices of subjective well-being, but the process and effects of institutional socialization weaken the credibility of subject's own reports of their inner feelings and state of mind. Part of the problem stems from the apathy induced by institutional life creating unthinking compliance as well as powerlessness and reliance on staff fostering a mood of quiescence and submissiveness. These are compounded by the fact that people's satisfactions are conditioned by their expectations (Runciman, 1966) and dependency may foster feelings of indebtedness and gratitude toward carers which cannot be taken as acceptance of either infirmity or other life circumstances. Psychological well-being is therefore not only a measure of response to care and the environment in which that care is received but encompasses feelings about those changes in circumstances, which have resulted in being cared for in an institution. As Booth writes, 'for some it is not so much a matter of whether the care they receive maximizes their subjective well being but whether it minimizes the damage they have suffered' (1985, p. 103).

Bearing these points in mind, it remains paramount in studies which purport to assess the effectiveness of care provision that appropriately constructed measures of personal well-being are included.

Quality Adjusted Life Years

In principle the outcome of any health care procedure can be measured in terms of their effect on life expectancy and quality of life. Measures of quality adjusted life years (QUALYs) were designed so that the outcome of health care procedures could be measured in a single index over time. The QUALY measure is a combination of expected life years gained from consumption of a health care procedure and some judgement (represented by an index) about the quality of life years gained. To date the approach has been used to measure the outcome of acute health care procedures (Williams, 1985) but in its current state of development is not viewed as practical in assessing the outcome of long-term care (Donaldson *et al.*, 1988).

Intermediate Outcomes

While we would regard subjective well-being as being of primary significance, there are other measurable outcomes which are associated with the quality of care provided and which are likely to influence the quality of life. These outcomes, which we have called intermediate outcomes, and which are defined principally by the behaviour of individuals, are likely to be in a reflexive relationship with different kinds of institutional regimes. The research problem is to tease out the nature of those relationships and the manner in which they influence individual behaviour.

Self-rated Health

Self-rated health has been used as a proxy measure for personal well-being but it is clearly in an antecedent relationship to personal well being. Measures of self-rated health have been shown to be predictive of survival (Kay et al., 1966) and of admission to an institution (Townsend, 1965). Changes in self-rated health following relocation have been found to vary with the degree of environmental change (Bourestom and Tars, 1974). Measures of self-rated health are reviewed by Davies and Knapp (1981). They are fairly straightforward to administer and often take a comparative approach by asking respondents to rate their health in relation to others.

Morbidity

Like self-rated health, morbidity is predictive of survival. Yet it remains a difficult dimension to measure, because a clinical diagnosis may reflect a variety of different health states. Although some attempts have been made to monitor changes in diagnoses (MacDonald et al., 1982) and relate them to different forms of care this approach has been seemingly unsuccessful particularly in the case of elderly people where any one individual may have a number of diagnoses attributed to them. The difficulties of detecting and interpreting changes in diagnoses has focused research on the effects of morbidity on behavioural functioning. Two groups of studies can be identified. Those in which some form of behaviour classification is undertaken and those which use tests of physical function.

Behaviour classifications have usually been based on reported behaviour. Two types are most common. First those which categorize individuals' capacities for activities of daily living (Akhtar et al., 1973; Bond and Carstairs, 1982; Clarke et al., 1979; Katz et al., 1970; Harris, Cox and Smith, 1971; McDowell, Martini and Waugh, 1978; Rosow and Breslau, 1966; Townsend, 1979; Townsend and Wedderburn, 1965) and second, those which categorize individuals on the basis of general levels of social functioning rather than specific activities of daily living (Gilleard and Pattie, 1977; Robinson, 1971; Wilkin, Mashiah and Jolley, 1978). The first group normally rely on information provided by subjects and the second group on information provided by professionals or close relatives about subjects.

A frequent problem encountered in behaviour classification is the distinction between ability and actual performance. A related difficulty is the differential perception of ability by the respondent and observers. Such problems highlight the complex relationship between a subject's perceptions of health state and final outcomes.

A few studies have used tests of physical function in which the subject is asked to perform simple tasks (Fitzpatrick and Donovan, 1979; Jefferys *et al.*, 1969; Katz *et al.*, 1962). Tests of physical function may provide a more reliable estimate of behavioural ability but they appear difficult to administer in anything but a clinical setting and abilities in one environment such as hospital do not necessarily equate with abilities in another environment such as a subject's own home.

In order to deal with the interacting effects of the behavioural abilities of individuals, the press of the environment, and the quality of prevailing relationships between subjects and their carers, the term dependency is often used as a short form to describe physical and psychological dependency.

Dependency

For many years the concept of dependency has continued to be an enigma. It has been used in so many ways that it is often difficult to ascertain its usefulness in the context of particular studies. Walker (1982) shows that the concept has been widely employed in at least four different ways: life-cycle dependency, physical and psychological dependency, political dependency and economic and financial dependency. Wilkin (1986) shows how the major emphasis has been on the concept of physical and psychological dependency, which we have called behavioural ability. The wider and more appropriate use of the term dependency can be explicated by considering the relationship between residents and staff in residential homes. Residents will not only be physically and psychologically dependent on staff because of physical and mental frailty but they will also be politically dependent in terms of the control they have over their own lives and financially dependent in terms of their dependence on state benefits. Thus dependency implies some kind of subordinate relationship between the dependent person and the people being depended on. In institutions residents are dependent on staff in all the ways characterized by Walker (1982).

Thus dependency in the general and the specific sense of physical and psychological dependency has been used frequently as an intermediate outcome. For example, Pattie, Gilleard and Bell (1979) studied a sample of people drawn from the community, local authority residential homes, geriatric wards and psychogeriatric wards over a two-year period. They found changes in the behavioural characteristics of survivors were slight irrespective of location. Using the same behaviour classification method Miller (1985) found differences in some components of the instrument, sufficient to provide an overall difference in behavioural characteristics with patients cared for in wards where individualized care was provided being less incapacitated than those where care was carried out on a 'task allocation' basis. While this was a cross-sectional study with no control, a comparison of the two care regimes in one ward showed a reduction in incapacity when individualized care planning was introduced. Unfortunately there was no detailed description of either types of nursing care.

In a study of ten old peoples' homes Townsend and Kimbell (1975) related information about the behavioural characteristics of the residents to the physical and social environmental characteristics of the homes in which they lived. While there was no overall relationship between measures of regime and behaviour classifications, there appeared to be less mental confusion in homes characterized as more personalized. The study design did not control for admissions policy and so it was not possible to say which came first.

A more thorough test of the 'induced dependency hypothesis' stated in the form that 'the more institutional regimes deny residents control over their own lives the more they tend to foster their dependency' (Booth, 1985, p. 129) was carried out in 178 local authority homes. It failed to show any relationship between type of institutional regime and outcome. While the homes studied were different according to the Institutional Regimes Questionnaire constructed to assess the dimensions of personal choice, privacy, segregation and participation, they were not sufficiently different to influence dependency. The observed differences in rates of improvement and deterioration among residents in different homes must have been attributable to factors other than those tapped.

Willcocks, Peace and Kellaher (1987) found that in old peoples' homes, those that offered greater opportunity for stimulation and activity showed a negative association with the proportion of mentally infirm residents, while the level of physical impairments was positively associated with staff-oriented environments.

The directness and sensitivity of the variety of measures used in these studies are undoubtedly influential in being able to tap differences, but the multifactorial nature of the process makes the establishment of direct cause–effect relationships improbable.

Type and Level of Activity

The last group of intermediate outcomes described concerns activity. While the activity theory of ageing (Havinghurst and Albrecht, 1953) proposes that continued levels of activity among elderly people promotes self-esteem and personal well-being, disengagement theory (Cumming and Henry, 1961) concludes that withdrawal and reduction in activity is advantageous. Advocates of activity theory like Kushlik and Blunden (1974) suggest that the old person's behaviour may itself be used as an index of care. An institution is providing *good* care if the clients are engaged in adaptive activity which indicates appropriate procedures are being used to maintain skills.

Godlove, Richard and Rodwell (1982) have compared activity levels of matched groups of old people being cared for in different care settings: day centres, local authority homes, day hospitals and hospital wards. Substantial variations were found which were not attributable to the subjects' behavioural abilities. Patients in hospital wards spent 72 per cent of their time doing nothing and talking to no one compared with 53 per cent in local authority homes, 40 per cent in day hospitals and 23 per cent in day centres. While overall levels of engagement in meaningful activity discriminates between different care settings (McFadyen, 1984), it does not follow that increased engagement means improved personal well-being (Townsend and Kimbell, 1975; Mercer and Kane, 1979). In the same way disengagement is open to different interpretations. There is little to choose between *enforced* activity and *enforced* inactivity. However, descriptive accounts of planned changes in the environment to deinstitutionalize it (Gupta, 1979) or unplanned changes (Adams, 1979) have shown spontaneous changes in activities and activity levels. Thus, while increased engagement *per se* does not ensure a better quality of life, when care is provided in a less institutionalized environment it is likely to result in more engagement and this may provide one contribution to an improved quality of life. As well as judging the efficacy of engagement on final outcomes within its environmental context, individual differences in the salience of engaged activity for quality of life require to be taken into account (Davies and Knapp, 1981).

Rather than examine amount of activity or engagement some inferences about quality of care can be drawn from examining patients behaviour in specific 'critical incidents'. Elliot (1975) has pointed out that mealtimes are often the highlight of an otherwise eventless day and so the manner in which meals are eaten are an important contribution to the patients quality of life. Davies and Snaith (1980a, b) have demonstrated that long-stay wards may be distinguished by the level and type of social interaction that occurs at lunchtime, by what staff regard as therapeutic and by the way that lunchtimes are organized. They found that it was possible, by changing seating arrangements and providing prompts, to increase social behaviour and allow patients to exert more control over the waythey ate.

Other studies using behavioural techniques have shown that it is possible to promote desirable behaviour like bathing (Rinke *et al.*, 1978), independent eating and mobility (Geiger and Johnson, 1974; Baltes and Zerbe, 1976) or reduce incontinence (Tarrier and Larner, 1983). Thus the ways that staff support dependence maintaining behaviours and ignore independent personal maintenance (Barton, Baltes and Orzech, 1980) affects residents level of functioning and consequent well-being. This relationship between staff practices and resident behaviours highlights that intermediate outcomes are contingent upon process.

Process

Physical Environment

How individuals cope in their physical environment will also influence their personal well-being. The 'environmental docility hypothesis' that 'the less competent the individual, the greater the impact of environmental factors on that individual' (Lawton, 1980, p. 14) includes physical as well as other dimensions of the environment. While environmental press may create sufficient stimulus for some individuals to experience growth it may also exert too few demands, leading to withdrawal and atrophy of adaptive behaviours. The physical environment can be viewed from both functional and symbolic perspectives; it can be regarded as fulfilling particular functions for those who use it but also as embodying particular ideologies. Poor-law workhouses, in which many elderly people are still cared for, are a clear testimony to the functional warehousing of Victorian benevolence.

We can assess whether long-stay intitutional environments cater for the needs of *residents* or staff or neither; to what degree domesticity is achievable with units of twenty or more people; and in what ways environmental arrangements influence functionally adaptive behaviour and social integration. Physical environments, like their social counterparts, can be analysed through different levels and across different dimensions. Architectural and physical design features, as well as furnishings and equipment, are included. Officials guidelines concerning the physical environment of hospital wards for old people (DHSS, 1981) and residential homes (DHSS *et al.*, 1973) are available and a basic level of analysis would relate the facilities available against these official standards. This poses the question of which aspects of these different building notes are most relevant to different kinds of long-stay accommodation for elderly people.

Aspects of the physical environment enhances or interferes with individual well-being in the way it influences, for example, privacy through the provision of not only space for solitude or intimacy with others but also anonymity in public spaces. Juxtaposed with public anonymity is the expression of territorial rights to particular spaces. The spatial arrangement of chairs in public sitting-rooms and the potential effects on sociability as well as privacy has been the subject of some debate (Lipman and Slater, 1977).

The physical environment also features in resident autonomy. Lawton (1970) comments that activities of daily living are more easily maintained if toilets, bathrooms and dining facilities are situated close to sitting areas. Finlay *et al.* (1983) demonstrated that adherence to guidelines on seating design influenced independent mobility and that staff were able to avoid a considerable amount of lifting. Space to permit mobility using wheelchairs and other aids also will influence autonomy. Personal autonomy extends to broader areas of life-style and to control over, for example, possessions and the immediate physical environment like opening and closing windows, or switching lights on and off. The ability to be autonomous will depend therefore on how prosthetic the environment has been made, but also on opportunities to exercise autonomy.

The mental capacity of many elderly people is such that orientation to physical locations may be impaired, especially when presented with complex spatial arrangements. Canter and Canter (1979) suggest that inability to form a mental picture of spatial locations leads to greater dependency, if not to total passivity. Thus, more complex buildings which lack adequate signposting, may limit activities and reinforce feelings of disorientation and confusion.

In designing appropriate physical environments there is a balancing of different forces, for example between providing furnishings and fabrics which are domestic and those which are easy to clean, or seating arrangements which foster sociability yet permit privacy. Nowhere is this idea of balancing more evident than in the realm of safety. Fire precautions influence the type of furnishings, the strength of door hinges and the rules governing where and when smoking is allowed. Whether residents can lock the door when using the toilet, bathroom or own bedroom is related to safety precautions. The spatial location of furniture and seating are associated with the risks of residents falling. However, excessive attention to safety serve to minimize risk taking and expressions of individuality and promote block treatment (Willcocks, Peace and Kellaher, 1987).

Avoidance of risks is also likely to influence the likelihood of residents going out and their involvement in the world beyond the confines of the institution. Rowles (1981) emphasizes the importance of visual contact with the world outside to positively facilitate adjustment to life in an institutional setting. For frail elderly people, the opportunity to 'watch the world go by' from within may be their major source of stimulation. Community integration involves, as well as the local community coming into the institution, residents and staff participating in life outside. The physical location of the institution within a community as well as the physical environment will therefore be an important influence on the personal well-being of residents.

Social Environment

Goldberg and Connelly conclude from their review of the extensive literature on social care that there appears to be little agreement about what characterizes good quality care for the very elderly. Nevertheless they construct a list of those features of the social environment which are currently held to influence life in social care homes for the better:

1 flexibility of management practices;
2 individualization and autonomy for residents;
3 opportunities for privacy;
4 opportunities for social stimulation;
5 communication and interaction with the outside world;
6 social interaction between staff and residents (in addition to instrumental communication);
7 maximum delegation of decision-making to care staff and to residents;
8 good communication channels between staff;
9 a minimum degree of specialization of roles and tasks among staff – (Goldberg and Connelly, 1982, pp. 272–3).

Dick (1985) has challenged nurses 'in ward or residential home' to consider whether some of these features exist, indicating the relevance of similar indices for both settings.

Attempts to conceptualize and measure different care environments derive from different purposes, focus on different features and assess them in different ways.

The work of Moos (Moos *et al.*, 1979) stems from the needs-press model of the relationship between environment and behaviour and has led to the development of a number of indices which attempt to measure the social environment of institutions. This model seeks to determine how people feel about where they are living by asking them to rate it on a number of different dimensions.

Using data from a large number of different types of institutions for elderly people Lemke and Moos (1986) construct eight indices which cover aspects of the structure and process of care and which may be used to depict the characteristics of an institution in comparison to normative data. These indices are characterized by the terms: comfort, security, staffing levels, staff richness, services, autonomy, control and rapport. The data show that these eight indices are only moderately interrelated, supporting the view that quality of care is multi-dimensional and that staffing levels are relatively independent of the other quality indices. This work also shows that different kinds of institutions characterized as nursing homes, residential homes or sheltered housing are reflected by differences in their scale scores on different dimensions and that scores also differ according to whether settings are proprietary or non-profit, and by their size. Nursing homes, for example, show less autonomy, provide a more protective environment with more security and services and higher staffing levels than other types of institutions examined.

This recent work by Moos changes the focus and extends his earlier work which was concerned solely with the social atmosphere of institutions and did not take account of other 'domains of environmental dimensions' which may influence social atmosphere. Physical and architectural features, policy and programme attributes and the characteristics of residents and staff are domains which were found to influence the social environment. These findings go some way towards identifying what factors or combination of factors make the same category of institution different; why some are 'better' than others; and what it is that causes some environments to make more demands on some individuals than others resulting in some residents being able to cope and others not.

A second approach to assessing institutional environments derives from the work of Pincus (Pincus, 1968; Pincus and Wood, 1970). Rather than focus on the subjective feelings of residents to discriminate between different kinds of environments, feelings which are influenced by the resident's functional health and other features of their situation, Pincus concentrates on participants' descriptions of the characteristics of their environment. Such characteristics include the physical features, the kinds of rules, regulations and programmes and staff behaviour with residents. It also differs from the approach used by Moos by omitting the intrapersonal characteristics of residents and interpersonal relationships between residents and between residents and staff.

Both of these approaches represent attempts to assess the social environments of an institution in broad terms, using a number of different dimensions. Another approach is to characterize the prevailing regime within an institution and this approach has been used within hospital wards as well as other types of institutions, including those for elderly people. Important in this respect is the work of Sinclair (1971) who identified the warden's attitude and approach to managing hostels for probationers led to differences in the attitudes of staff and the existing regime. He argues that the success of 'quasi-family' institutions, such as probation hostels depends more on the quality of the relationships than on rules and routines (Sinclair, 1971). This approach has been extended by Cawson and Perry (1977) to schools where they developed a measure of staff attitudes towards the style of control they felt should be adopted and the style of relationship which they felt they should have with the boys. The attitudes of staff on these aspects of regime were shown to be related to the behaviour of children in residential settings (Martin, 1977).

Studies in hospitals have focused on the ward sister's role (Pembrey, 1980; Runciman, 1983) as being crucial to how wards are organized but studies are not yet forthcoming on whether this influences outcomes for patients. Baker (1978) demonstrated in geriatric wards how prevailing attitudes of rank and file staff toward both their work and their patients can overwhelm the effects of a ward sister who showed markedly positive attitudes to individualized humanitarian care, so that care remains routinized and impersonalized, with an emphasis on 'getting through and getting straight'. Those who attempted to deviate from this style of nursing regarded their patients as 'whole and usual persons'. 'Routine geriatric' style is perpetrated, however, where wards and their personnel are physically and socially isolated and they perceive status denial by such things as few resources, both material and non-material, and the unimportance attached to long-stay wards in both the geriatric unit and the hospital. This reinforces Sinclair's finding that the attitude of the person in charge could be influential so long as other structural characteristics of the institution permitted it. Baker shows that characteristics of hospitals may overwhelm the influence of a ward sister in a geriatric ward to produce a particular care regime.

The term 'care' is itself open to a host of interpretations and finds expression at a number of levels, cross cut by profession and other interests. For example, Wade, Sawyer and Bell (1983) found differential levels of medication in different care settings, with the lowest levels in voluntary and private residential homes and the highest levels in private nursing homes. Hospital patients received more laxatives while patients in private nursing homes received most psychotropic medication. This kind of evidence suggests that patients under different medical regimes may receive differential types and levels of medication, with consequent effects on their health status and level of functioning.

The care of old people will be influenced by particular ideologies which legitimize the prevalent care regime whatever the kind of institution. In a study of eight geriatric wards Evers (1981) characterized care regimes as minimal warehousing or personalized warehousing and found that the ward sister's scheduling of work and the structure of the relationship between the ward sister and the consultant determined the categorization used. Ward sisters who created care characterized by personal warehousing organized care at least partially on a patient-centred basis and patient care was explicitly defined as valid and valuable by the doctors who acknowledged this by their behaviour. In contrast, in wards where sisters did not organize care on a patient-centred basis, and where minimal warehousing characterized the mode of care, the consultants defined caring for patients as less important than cure and this was expressed verbally and by their behaviour. While these findings conjure a depressing picture of the hospital careers of long-stay patients, they are consonant with other nursing studies (Baker, 1978; Wells, 1980). More recently Miller (1985) has attempted to characterize nursing care as individualized or task allocation.

Studies which have attempted to characterize the care regime are closely related to attempts to measure different aspects of the social environment. For example, King and Raynes (1968) developed a scale comprising four dimensions which distinguish practices in institutions for mentally-handicapped children which are 'institution oriented' from those which are 'inmate oriented'. More recently similar approaches have been used to assess the physical and organizational aspects of care in institutions for elderly people (Evans *et al.*, 1981; Wade, Sawyer and

Bell, 1983; Booth, 1985; Willcocks, Peace and Kellaher 1987). However, when comparing the social characteristics of residential homes, Willcocks and her colleagues and Booth both found that differences *between* homes in the way they are run are more than matched by differences *within* homes. Both studies show that homes demonstrate policies which seem to pull in different directions and they perform differently in sub-scales assessing their regime. While differences exist between homes, Willcocks, Peace and Kellaher conclude that 'we are still left with an overall impression supported by our observations, that residential life, whatever the setting, is predominantly public and communal, routinised and impersonal' (1987, p. 121). The question for us is whether life in hospital is any different from nursing-home life. Wade, Sawyer and Bell (1983) found the social environment even more institutional in long-stay hospital wards than in residential homes like those studied by Booth and Willcocks *et al.*, whereas private nursing homes were more personalized and democratic.

Quality of Working Life

It could be hypothesized that a satisfied staff is more likely to contribute to positive resident well-being than not. There is a counter argument, however, that a staff group which is organization oriented and which is relatively self-contained and self-centred will work to the detriment, if not the neglect of resident well-being (Willcocks, Peace and Kellaher, 1987). Thus there is no simple relationship between how staff regard the quality of their working life and the quality of resident well-being.

The assessment of the quality of working life is not straight forward and there are no universally accepted methods. A synthetic approach to assessing job satisfaction like that advocated by Cope (1981) would contain elements of discrepancy theories, equity theories and expectancy theories. Using a multidimensional scale Wallace and Cope (1980) found that despite many protestations of frustration and complaint regarding the features of their work in a psychogeriatric ward, many nursing staff expressed a high degree of overall satisfaction with their job. The satisfying elements included keeping busy, the appeal of doing things with other people, social relationships with other staff, having good supervisors, doing work which was on the whole interesting, having a fair amount of variety and getting at least an occasional feeling of achievement. Those elements which were bad clustered around working conditions and amenities, particularly alleged staff shortages resulting in inadequate care; inadequate consultation and lack of involvement in decisions; and inadequacies in their training. These nurses worked in a system of care which generated high anxiety, uncertainty of purpose and fostered institutionalization, was regarded as low status, yet they displayed high levels of job satisfaction. These findings are similar to White's (1980) in American long-term nursing homes.

Comparing levels of job satisfaction in social care homes, Willcocks, Peace and Kellaher (1987) found the lowest levels in homes where there was below average staff hours to residents. This was particularly so in relation to perceived job autonomy where working methods and variety were likely to be restricted and time allowed only the essentials of care to be tackled. Enhanced job satisfaction was associated with higher numbers of part-time staff as well as higher numbers of staff hours per resident. The satisfaction staff obtained was in part due to this capacity to organize and control the demands made upon them. There are obvious interrelationships here with management practices and other features of the social environment in which staff work.

Structure

Attitudes of Staff

The attitudes of staff affect not only their own expectations about their working lives but also the way in which they approach residents. Social attitudes stereotype elderly people leading to ageism, which may be reflected in the care elderly people receive and may influence society's response to the kind of care deemed appropriate and to that provided by professionals. This was certainly the case in the geriatric wards studied by Baker (1978) where patients were regarded as child like, unreliable and manipulative with the resulting emphasis given to depersonalizing physical care and the neglect of psychosocial needs.

Fielding (1986) examined student nurses' accounts of their interactions with elderly people and found a tendency to attribute dependency, mental confusion and inability for self-care to old age. Attitudes are the product of socialization and Fielding suggests that the experiences student nurses met during their education will do little to change their attitudes for the better. This has implications for those who will ultimately provide care.

Organizational Structure and Policy

The prevailing social environment in an institution is embedded within and influenced by wider organizational relationships. One way of looking at organizational arrangements is along bureaucratic dimensions, of which Raynes, Pratt and Roses (1979) identified four: centralisation, formalization, communication and specialization. Centralization concerns the extent to which authority is delegated. Formalization describes the extent to which rules and regulations constrain the manner in which tasks are carried out by workers. Communication refers to the level of contact staff have with other groups involved in resident care and specialization identifies the degree to which the task of caring is divided between tasks which are shared by staff.

Raynes *et al.* suggested that together ratings on these dimensions of homes for mentally-handicapped children was associated with the prevailing regime. Evers (1982) in describing the influence of organizational structure on patient care in geriatric wards found that low levels of teamwork was associated with high specialization and low communication between different professional groups. Wells (1980) also noted the centralization and formalization in hospitals resulting in authoritarianism and institutionalism with an absence of personalized concern for staff and patients alike. Clearly then, organizational structure has a bearing on both the quality of working life for staff and the quality of care of residents.

Staff Inputs

A major input affecting the quality of care of residents is the number and quality of staff. Yet we are devoid of studies which examine this relationship. Most attempts have been devoted to establishing staffing requirements for particular groups of clients (Senior, 1978) or in accordance with prescribed tasks (Rhys-Hearn, 1979) without regard for the quality of care or its outcome. When nursing staff were allocated in accordance with nurses' identification of patients' optimal nursing requirements, Rhys-Hearn (1979) found that in no case was the care given equivalent to the care prescribed. Norwich (1980) noted that when 'extra' time was available it was spent in physical care activities rather than psycho-social or therapeutic support, a finding supported by Savage, Widdowson and Wright (1979) about psychogeriatric wards. Since under usual circumstances nurses adjust their work practices to enable them to complete the work they regard as essential, it is not surprising that there is little change in the type of work carried out with temporarily increased staff. Even if more time is spent on physical care, Evans *et al.* (1981) found in social-care homes that social aspects of care are not embedded in physical assistance to bathe and such like.

The available staff hours per resident may not be as important as the type of staff. Willcocks, Peace and Kellaher (1987) found that senior staff in social-care homes had more resident-oriented views on features of residential life while care staff were more likely to express views that spring from organizational needs for routine. Since ideas about care provision are likely to flow from senior staff, then available hours and organizational practices which permit them to demonstrate skilled care and supervise care staff are necessary. Otherwise they only carry out inspection to ensure the worst practices are avoided.

Willcocks, Peace and Kellaher also found that staff-oriented rather than resident-oriented practices were strongest in homes with the lowest staffing levels. Staff shortages resulted in dispensing with flexibility for both residents and staff with formalization of the care regime in order to complete what was regarded as essential work. Homes with higher staff : resident hours and a higher proportion of part-time staff rather than full-time staff were more likely to have resident-oriented practices as well as higher levels of agreement between staff and residents about what constitutes ideal environmental features.

The reciprocal relationship between quality of care and levels of staff turnover has been referred to since Revans (1964) found that high turnover of nurses in acute hospitals was related to length of patient stay. Garibaldi, Brodine and Matsumiya (1981) found the physical care of nursing-home residents in the USA deteriorated during high staff turnover and Stryker (1981) hypothesizes that depression, disengagement, disorientation and isolation among long-term residents is likely to increase when staff–resident relationships are disrupted by high turnover. Thus the staff hours available, the relationships between full-time and part-time staff and staff turnover are likely to be relevant to the quality of care.

Staff Knowledge

Traditionally, changes to staff education have featured as policy recommendations for changing nursing practice and nurses' attitudes. But does the level of knowledge among staff influence nursing practice and hence resident outcomes? Wells (1980), in her study of nurses working on geriatric wards in the early 1970s, found that the study nurses lacked knowledge and skill. Wells attributed this to a training system which taught them a series of tasks and neglected to provide them with adequate information about patient care, resulting in ritualistic routines without regard for their consequences.

Fielding (1986) studying nursing students found that students tended neither to expect to enjoy nor did enjoy nursing geriatric patients, regarding it as 'boring' and physically taxing, while offering little valuable experience. Their experience was embedded within an education system which had failed to indicate any specific role for nurses to play but which had spelled out the contribution of other professionals. Such formal guidance as 'letting the patient help themselves' in the absence of specific nursing assessments and care planning results in care which students themselves describe as 'too routine', 'monotonous' and that 'nothing happened'.

Of course, student nurses are a minor and transient component of the staffing of geriatric units, and knowledge of geriatric care should reside in the permanent qualified staff. It was not until 1979, however, that a component of geriatric nursing became compulsory in the training of British student nurses.

More recently, Kitson (1984) has shown in a study of ward sisters that they could be distributed along a dimension of perceived therapeutic nursing function. Low scores defined geriatric nursing as 'just basic nursing care' and 'hard work', the physical maintenance of patients and carrying out medical objectives. Assessment of patients' needs was sketchy with no clear system of collecting or utilizing patient information. They perceived their training needs as limited. By comparison high scorers felt a need for additional education and showed more detailed knowledge of nurses' contribution to the goal of achieving optimal independence. They also had a more sharply focused idea of the nurses' role in contributing to the rehabilitation process in patient care. In order to be a high scorer a sophisticated skill repertoire was necessary which was grounded in a theoretical framework and practised in an individualized way.

Evaluating Long-term Care

In this chapter we have attempted to review the state of the art in evaluating long-term care for elderly people. In so doing we have found it necessary to relate this description to the changing social policies about the care of elderly people in modern Britain. Thus this chapter has two major themes and hence a title emphasizing trends in development and evaluation. Both these themes are changing. We have shown how changes in the population structure, political ideologies and the objectives of geriatric medicine have influenced the kinds of care provided by doctors, nurses, social workers and other professional groups. We have highlighted broad changes in perspectives adopted in the evaluation of long-term care and described appropriate studies within the broad framework of a model of evaluation developed from the social welfare perspective used in the evaluation of residential care. Necessarily the chapter is incomplete and provides a summary statement, which only hints at the complexity of methodological issues involved.

The approach taken to evaluating long-term care has been influenced by the academic disciplinary and professional experiences of the authors together with colleagues involved in a study to evaluate long-stay accommodation for elderly people with a particular interest in the three experimental NHS nursing homes. This has brought a social science and nursing focus to the chapter, although not exclusively so.

From this review we would suggest that there is, in line with other areas of nursing, an absence of a well-developed body of nursing knowledge. As we have indicated, the majority of nursing studies are small scale and descriptive. Irrespective of discipline, there are few controlled evaluative studies of long-term institutional care, although there are now a small number of useful large-scale descriptive studies of residential care. British studies of nursing-home care, and of all private care, are particularly lacking and this concerns us, given the expansion of this type of care in recent years.

We would conclude that evaluating long-term care for elderly people requires both multiple perspectives and multiple methods. These perspectives and methods should be seen as complementary rather than competing. Traditional single-perspective approaches using a standard single method are too limiting, leaving many questions unanswered and providing no justifiable prescription for action. Studies which are multi-perspective tend to attempt to answer a range of questions and use a variety of methods to do so. They are not without problems but are more informative. A fundamental feature of such evaluation studies should be the opportunity for controlled comparisons, for without well-controlled outcome studies, policy-makers will be unable to make informed judgements about the efficacy of different approaches to long-term care. However, an important feature of such studies would also be a description of the structures and processes which influence outcomes. Without such descriptions it would be difficult to replicate a method of care to produce the desirable outcomes. The model we have described is not complete and will evolve over the next few years, being informed by our present work, and the numerous research endeavours which are currently in progress throughout the world.

Acknowledgement

We are grateful for financial support from DHSS and to colleagues in the Health Care Research Unit, particularly Cam Donaldson for his ideas on quality adjusted life years and Freda Bolam and Eva Brown for their help in the preparation of this chapter.

References

Adams, G. F. (1952). Long-stay accommodation for the elderly irremediable patient, *Ulster Medical Journal*, **xxi**, 177–184.
Adams, G. F. (1964). Clinical undertaking? *Lancet*, **ii**, 1055–1058.
Adams, J. (1979). A change of scene: 1 Ridge Hill, or home not a ward: features of the bungalow. *Nursing Times*, **75** (39), 1659–1661.
Akhtar, A. J., Broe, G. A., Crombie, A., McLean, W. M. R., Andrews, G. R. and Caird, F. I. (1973). Disability and dependence in the elderly at home. *Age and Ageing*, **2**, 102–111.
Alexander, J. R. and Eldon, A. (1979). Characteristics of elderly people admitted to hospital, Part III homes, and sheltered housing. *Epidemiology and Community Health*, **33**, 91–95.
Andrews, G. R., Cowan, N. R. and Anderson, W. F. (1971). The practice of geriatric medicine in the community, in McLachlan (Ed.), *Problems and Progress in Medical Care*, Fifth Series, pp. 57–86. Oxford University Press, London.
Atkinson, D. A., Bond, J. and Gregson, B. A. (1986). The dependency characteristics of older people in long term institutional care, in C. Phillipson, M. Bernard and P. Strang (Eds), *Dependency and Interdependency in Old Age — Theoretical Perspectives and Policy Alternatives*, pp. 257–269. Croom Helm, London.
Baker, D. E. (1978). *Attitudes of nurses to the care of the elderly*. Unpublished PhD Thesis, University of Manchester.
Baltes, M. M. and Zerbe, M. B. (1976). Independence training in the nursing home resident. *The Gerontologist*, **26**, 428–432.
Barnes, C. (1980). *The Relentless Tide: A Study of Admissions into Homes for the Elderly*. Social Services Department, Training and Development Division, Surrey County Council.
Barton, E. M., Baltes, M. M. and Orzech, M. J. (1980). Aetiology of dependents in older nursing home residents during morning care: the role of staff behaviour. *Journal of Personality and Social Psychology*, **38**, 423–431.
Bebbington, A. and Tong, M. (1983). Trends and changes in old people's homes: provision over 20 years, in *Seminar on Residential Care for Elderly People: Background Papers and Synopses of Research*. DHSS, London.
Bergmann, K., Foster, E. M., Justice, A. W. and Matthews, V. (1978). Management of the demented elderly patient in the community. *British Journal of Psychiatry*, **132**, 441–449.
Berkeley, J. S. (1976). Reasons for referral to hospital. *Journal of the Royal College of General Practitioners*, **26**, 293–296.

Blessed, G. and Wilson, D. (1982). The contemporary natural history of mental disorder in old age. *British Journal of Psychiatry*, **141**, 59–67.

Bond, J. (1984). Evaluation of long-stay accommodation for elderly people, in D. B. Bromley (Ed.), *Gerontology: Social and Behavioural Perspectives*, pp. 88–101. Croom Helm, London.

Bond, J. (1987) Psychiatric illness in later life. A study of prevalence in a Scottish population. *International Journal of Geriatric Psychiatry*, **2**, 39–58.

Bond, J. and Carstairs, V. (1982). *Services for the Elderly: A Survey of the Characteristics and Needs of a Population of 5,000 Old People*. Scottish Health Service Studies No. 42. Scottish Home and Health Department, Edinburgh.

Booth, T. (1985). *Home Truths. Old People's Homes and the Outcome of Care*. Gower, Aldershot.

Booth, T. and Phillips, D. with Barritt, A., Berry, S., Martin, D. N. and Melotte, C. (1983). A follow-up study of trends in dependency in local authority homes for the elderly 1980–82. *Research Policy and Planning*, **1**, 1–9.

Bourestom, N. and Tars, S. (1974). Alterations in life patterns following nursing home relocation. *The Gerontologist*, **14**, 506–510.

Bradburn, N. M. (1969). *The Structure of Psychological Well-being*. Aldine, Chicago, Ill.

Brauer, E., Mackeprang, B. and Bentzon, M. W. (1978). Prognosis of survival in a geriatric population. *Scandinavian Journal of Social Medicine*, **6**, 17–24.

Brocklehurst, J. C. (Ed.) (1975). *Geriatric Care in Advanced Societies*. MTP, Lancaster.

Brocklehurst, J. C. (1978). Geriatric services and the day hospital, in J. C. Brocklehurst (Ed.) *Text Book of Geriatric Medicine and Gerontology*, Second Ed, pp. 747–762. Churchill Livingstone, Edinburgh.

Brocklehurst, J. C. and Andrews, K. (1985). Geriatric medicine — the style of practise. *Age and Ageing*, **14**, 1–7.

Brocklehurst, J. C., Carty, M. H., Leeming, J. T. and Robinson, J. M. (1978). Medical screening of old people accepted for residential care. *Lancet*, **ii**, 141–143.

Brocklehurst, J. C., Morris, P., Andrews, K., Richards, B. and Laycock, P. (1981). Social effects of stroke. *Social Science and Medicine*, **15A**, 35–39.

Canter, D. and Canter, S. (Eds) (1979). *Designing for Therapeutic Environments: A Review of Research*. John Wiley, Chichester.

Carstairs, V. and Morison, M. (1971). *The Elderly in Residential Care. Report of a Survey of Homes and their Residents*. Scottish Health Service Studies No. 19, Scottish Home and Health Department, Edinburgh.

Cartwright, A., Hockey, L. and Anderson, J. (1973). *Life Before Death*, Routledge & Kegan Paul, London.

Cawson, P. and Perry, J. (1977). Environmental correlates of attitude among residential staff. *British Journal of Criminology*, **17**, 141–156.

Charlesworth, A. and Wilkin, D. (1982). *Dependency among Old People in Geriatric Wards, Psychogeriatric Wards and Residential Homes 1977–1981*. Research Report No. 6. Departments of Psychiatry and Community Medicine, University of Manchester.

Charlesworth, A., Wilkin, D. and Durie, A. (1984). *Carers and Services: A*

Comparison of Men and Women Caring for Dependent Elderly People. Equal Opportunities Commission, Manchester.

Christie, A. B. (1982). Changing patterns in mental illness in the elderly. *British Journal of Psychiatry*, **140**, 154–159.

Clarke, M., Hughes, A. O., Dodd, K. J., Palmer, R. L., Brandon, S., Holden, A. M. and Pearce, D. (1979). The elderly in residential care: patterns of disability. *Health Trends*, **11**, 17–20.

Coid, J. and Crome, P. (1986). Bed blocking in Bromley. *British Medical Journal*, **292**, 1253–1256.

Cope, D. E. (1981). *Organisation Development and Action Research in Hospitals*. Gower, Aldershot.

Copeland, J. R. M., Kelleher, M. J., Kellett, J. M., Barron, G., Cowan, D. W. and Gourlay, A. J. (1975). Evaluation of a psychogeriatric service: the distinction between psychogeriatric and geriatric patients. *British Journal of Psychiatry*, **126**, 21–29.

Covell, B. and Angus, M. M. (1980). A comparison of the characteristics of elderly patients admitted to acute medical and geriatric wards. *Health Bulletin*, **38**, 64–70.

Cresswell, J. and Pasker, P. (1972). The frail who lead the frail. *New Society*, **20** (504), 407–410.

Cumming, E. and Henry, W. E. (1961). *Growing Old: The Process of Disengagement*. Basic Books, New York.

Currie, C. T., Smith, R. G. and Williamson, J. (1979). Medical and nursing needs of elderly patients admitted to acute medical beds. *Age and Ageing*, **8**, 149–151.

Davies, A. D. M. and Snaith, P. A. (1980a). Mealtime problems in a continuing care hospital for the elderly. *Age and Ageing*, **9**, 100–105.

Davies, A. D. M. and Snaith, P. A. (1980b). The social behaviour of geriatric patients at mealtimes: an observational and interventional study. *Age and Ageing*, **9**, 93–99.

Davies, B. and Knapp, M. (1981). *Old People's Homes and the Production of Welfare*, Routledge & Kegan Paul, London.

Davies, B. P., Barton, A. J., McMillan, I. S. and Williamson, V. K. (1971). *Variations in Services for the Aged. A Causal Analysis*, Occasional Papers on Social Administration, No. 40, Bell and Son, London.

Department of Health and Social Security and Welsh Office (1973). *Residential Accommodation for Elderly People*. Local Authority Building Note No. 2, HMSO, London.

Department of Health and Social Security (1981). *Hospital Accommodation for Elderly People*. Health Building Note 37. HMSO, London.

Department of Health and Social Security (1982). *Ageing in the United Kingdom*. DHSS, London.

Department of Health and Social Security (1983). *The Experimental National Health Service Nursing Homes for Elderly People. An Outline*. DHSS, London.

Dick, D. (1985). The institutional trap. *Nursing Times*, **81** (34), 47–48.

Dodd, K., Holden, A. and Reed, C. (1979). A census of elderly people in care. *Social Work Today*, **10**, 10–13.

Donabedian, A. (1980). *The Definition of Quality and Approaches to its Assessment*. Health Administration Press, Ann Arbor, Michigan.

Donaldson, C., Atkinson, D. A., Bond, J. and Wright, K. (1988). Quality adjusted life years in long-term care of elderly people. *Forthcoming*.

Donaldson, L. J., Clayton, D. G. and Clarke, M. (1980). The elderly in residential care: mortality in relation to functional capacity. *Journal of Epidemiology and Community Health*, **34**, 96–101.

Donaldson, L. J. and Jagger, C. (1983). Survival and functional capacity: three year follow up of an elderly population in hospitals and homes. *Journal of Epidemiology and Community Health*, **37**, 176–179.

Droller, H. (1969). Does community care really reach the elderly sick? *Gerontologia Clinica*, **ii**, 169–182.

Elliott, J. R. (1975). *Living in Hospital: The Social Needs of People in Long Term Care*. King Edward's Hospital Fund, London.

Equal Opportunities Commission (1980). *The Experience of Caring for Elderly and Handicapped Dependants: Survey Report*. Equal Opportunities Commission, Manchester.

Evans, G. J., Hodkinson, H. M. and Mezey, A. G. (1971). The elderly sick: who looks after them. *The Lancet*, **iii**, 539–541.

Evans, G., Hughes, B., Wilkin, D. and Jolley, D. (1981). *The Management of Mental and Physical Impairment in Non-specialist Residential Homes for the Elderly*. Research Report No. 4, Departments of Psychiatry and Community Medicine, University of Manchester, Manchester.

Evans, J. G. (1984). Prevention of age-associated loss of autonomy: epidemiological approaches. *Journal of Chronic Diseases*, **37**, 353–363.

Evers, H. K. (1981). The creation of patient careers in geriatric wards: aspects of policy and practice. *Social Science and Medicine*, **15A**, 581–588.

Evers, H. (1982). Professional practice and patient care: multi-disciplinary teamwork in geriatric wards. *Ageing and Society*, **2**, 57–75.

Farrow, S. C., Rablen, M. R. and Silver, C. P. (1976). Geriatric admissions in East London, 1962–1972. *Age and Ageing*, **5**, 49–55.

Fielding, P. (1986). *Attitudes Revisited: An Examination of Student Nurses' Attitudes Towards Old People in Hospital*. Royal College of Nursing, London.

Finch, J. and Groves, D. (Eds) (1983). *A Labour of Love: Women, Work and Caring*, Routledge & Kegan Paul, London.

Finlay, O. E., Bayles, T. B., Rosen, C. and Milling, J. (1983). Effects of chair design, age and cognitive status on mobility. *Age and Ageing*, **12**, 329–335.

Fitzpatrick, J. J. and Donovan, M. J. (1979). A follow-up study of the reliability and validity of the Motor Activity Rating Scale. *Nursing Research*, **28**, 179–181.

Foster, E. M., Kay, D. W. K. and Bergmann, K. (1976). The characteristics of old people receiving and needing domiciliary services: the relevance of psychiatric diagnosis. *Age and Ageing*, **5**, 245–255.

Gardiner, R. (1975). The identification of the medical and social needs of the elderly in the community: a pilot survey. *Age and Ageing*, **4**, 181–187.

Garibaldi, R. A., Brodine, R. N. and Matsumiya, R. N. (1981). Infections among patients in nursing homes. *New England Journal of Medicine*, **305**, 731–735.

Gedling, P. and Newell, D. J. (1972). Hospital beds for the elderly, in G.

McLachlan (Ed.) *Problems and Progress in Medical Care*, Sixth Series, pp. 133–145. Oxford University Press, Oxford.

Geiger, O. C. and Johnson, L. S. (1974). Positive education for elderly persons: correct eating through reinforcement. *Gerontologist*, **14**, 432–436.

Gilleard, C. J. (1980). Prevalence of incontinence in local authority homes for the elderly. *Health Bulletin*, **38**, 236–238.

Gilleard, C. J. and Pattie, A. H. (1977). The Stockton Geriatric Rating Scale: a shortened version with British normative data. *British Journal of Psychiatry*, **131**, 90–94.

Gilleard, C. J., Pattie, A. H. and Dearman, G. (1980). Behavioural disabilities in psychogeriatric patients and residents of old people's homes. *Journal of Epidemiology and Community Health*, **34**, 106–110.

Godlove, C., Richard, L. and Rodwell, G. (1982). *Time for Action. An Observation Study of Elderly People in Four Different Care Environments*. Joint Unit for Social Services Research, University of Sheffield.

Goffman, E. (1961). *Asylums: Essays on the Social Situation of Mental Patients and Other Inmates*. Anchor, New York.

Goldberg, E. M. and Connelly, N. (1982). *The Effectiveness of Social Care for the Elderly*. Heinemann, London.

Goldfarb, A. I. (1969). Predicting mortality in the institutionalised aged. *Archives of General Psychiatry*, **21**, 172–176.

Grad, J. and Sainsbury, P. (1968). The effects that patients have on their families in a community care and a central psychiatric service — a two year follow up. *British Journal of Psychiatry*, **508**, 265–278.

Graham, H. and Livesley, B. (1983). Can re-admission to a geriatric medical unit be prevented? *The Lancet*, **i**, 404–406.

Gruer, R. (1975). *Needs of the Elderly in the Scottish Borders*. Scottish Health Service Studies No. 33. Scottish Home and Health Department, Edinburgh.

Gupta, H. (1979). Can we de-institutionalise an institution? *Concord*, **13**, 47–57.

Halliburton, P. M. and Wright, W. B. (1974). Towards better geriatric care. *Social Work Today*, **5**, 107–108.

Harris, A. I. (1968). *Social Welfare for the Elderly*. Government Social Survey No. SS366. HMSO, London.

Harris, A. I., Cox, E. and Smith, C. R. W. (1971). *Handicapped and Impaired in Great Britain Part 1*. HMSO, London.

Havighurst, R. J. and Albrecht, R. (1953). *Older People*. Longman, London.

Hodkinson, H. M. (1981). *An Outline of Geriatrics*. Academic Press, London.

Hodkinson, H. M. and Hodkinson, I. (1980). Death and discharge from a geriatric department. *Age and Ageing*, **9**, 220–228.

Hodkinson, H. M., Evans, G. J. and Mezey, A. G. (1972). Factors associated with the misplacement of elderly patients in geriatric and psychiatric hospitals. *Gerontologia Clinica*, **14**, 267–273.

Hoenig, J. and Hamilton, M. W. (1966). Elderly psychiatric patients and the burden on the household. *Psychiatrica Neurologica*, **152**, 281–293.

Hunt, A. (1970). *The Home Help Service in England and Wales*. HMSO, London.

Illsley, R. (1980). *Professional or Public Health? Sociology in Health and Medicine*. Nuffield Provincial Hospitals Trust, London.

Isaacs, B. (1971). Geriatric patients: do their families care? *British Medical Journal*, **4**, 282–286.

Isaacs, B., Livingstone, M. and Neville, Y. (1972). *Survival of the Unfittest: A Study of Geriatric Patients In Glasgow*. Routledge & Kegan Paul, London.

Isaacs, B. and Neville, Y. (1975). *The Measurement of Need in Old People*. Scottish Health Service Studies No. 34. Scottish Home and Health Department, Edinburgh.

Jefferys, M., Millard, J. B., Hyman, M. and Warren, M. D. (1969). A set of tests for measuring motor impairment in prevalence studies. *Journal of Chronic Diseases*, **22**, 303–319.

Jones, D. A. and Vetter, N. J. (1984). A survey of those who care for the elderly at home: their problems and their needs. *Social Science and Medicine*, **19**, 511–514.

Katz, S., Downs, T. D., Cash, R. and Grotz, R. C. (1970). Progress in the development of the index of ADL. *The Gerontologist*, **10**, 20–30.

Katz, S., Jackson, B. A., Jaffe, M. W., Littell, A. S. and Turk, C. E. (1962). Multidisciplinary studies of illness in aged persons — VI. *Journal of Chronic Diseases*, **15**, 979–984.

Kay, D. W. K., Bergmann, K., Foster, E. and Garside, R. S. (1966). A 4-year follow-up of a random sample of old people originally seen in their homes. A physical, social and psychiatric enquiry. *Proceedings of the IV Congress of Psychiatry*, No. 150, 1668–1670.

Kidd, C. B. (1962). Misplacement of the elderly in hospital. *British Medical Journal*, **4**, 1491–1495.

King, R. D. and Raynes, N. V. (1968). An operational measure of inmate management in residential institutions. *Social Science and Medicine*, **2**, 41–53.

Kitson, A. L. (1984). Steps toward the identification and development of nursing's therapeutic function in the care of the hospitalised elderly. Unpublished PhD thesis, The New University of Ulster.

Kushlick, A. and Blunden, R. (1974). *Proposals for Setting up and Evaluation of an Experimental Service for the Elderly*. Research Report 107. Health Care Evaluation Research Team, Winchester.

Langley, E. E. and Simpson, J. H. (1970). Misplacement of the elderly in geriatric and psychiatric hospitals. *Gerontologia Clinica*, **12**, 149–163.

Lawton, M. P. (1970). Institutions for the aged: theory, content and methods for research. *The Gerontologist*, **10**, 305–312.

Lawton, M. P. (1972). The dimensions of morale, in D. P. Kent *et al.* (Eds), *Research Planning and Action for the Elderly*. Behavioural Publications, New York.

Lawton, M. P. (1975). The PGC Morale Scale: a revision. *Journal of Gerontology*, **30**, 85–89.

Lawton, M. P. (1980). *Environment and Aging*. Brooks/Cole Publishing Co., Monterey, California.

Lemke, S. and Moos, R. H. (1986). Quality of residential settings for elderly adults. *Journal of Gerontology*, **41**, 268–276.

Lipman, A. and Slater, R. (1977). Status and spacial appropriation in eight homes for old people. *Gerontologist*, **17**, 250–255.

Luker, K. A. (1979). Measuring life satisfaction in an elderly female population. *Journal of Advanced Nursing*, **4**, 503–511.

MacDonald, A. J. D., Mann, A. H., Jenkins, R., Richard, L., Godlove, C. and Rodwell, G. (1982). An attempt to determine the impact of four types of care upon the elderly in London by the study of matched groups. *Psychological Medicine*, **12**, 193–200.

Mann, A. H., Graham, N. and Ashby, D. (1984). Psychiatric illness in residential homes for the elderly: a survey on one London borough. *Age and Ageing*, **13**, 257–265.

Marks, J. (1975). *Home Help*. Bell & Sons, London.

Martin, D. N. (1977). Disruptive behaviour and staff attitudes at the St. Charles youth treatment centre. *Child Psychology and Psychiatry*, **18**, 221–228.

Masterton, G., Holloway, E. M. and Timbury, G. C. (1981). Role of local authority homes in the care of the dependent elderly: a prospective study. *British Medical Journal*, **283**, 523–524.

McArdle, C., Wylie, J. C. and Alexander, W. D. (1975). Geriatric patients in an acute medical ward. *British Medical Journal*, **4**, 568–569.

McDowell, I. W., Martini, C. J. and Waugh, W. (1978). A method for self-assessment of disability before and after hip replacement operations. *British Medical Journal*, **2**, 857–859.

McFadyen, M. (1984). The measurement of engagement in the institutionalised elderly, in I. Hanley and J. Hodge (Eds), *Psychological Approaches to the Care of the Elderly*, pp. 136–163. Croom Helm, London.

McKechnie, A. A. (1972). A point prevalence study of a long term hospital population. *Health Bulletin*, **xxxi**, 250–258.

McKeown, T. and Cross, K. W. (1969). Responsibilities of hospitals and local authorities for elderly patients. *British Journal of Preventive and Social Medicine*, **23**, 34–39.

McLauchlan, S. and Wilkin, D. (1982). Levels of provision and of dependency in residential homes for the elderly: implications for planning. *Health Trends*, **14**, 63–65.

Mercer, S. and Kane, R. A. (1979). Helplessness and hopelessness among the institutionalised aged: an experiment. *Health and Social Work*, **4**, 91–116.

Miller, A. (1985). A study of the dependency of elderly patients in wards using different methods of nursing care. *Age and Ageing*, **14**, 132–138.

Miller, E. J. and Gwynne, G. V. (1972). *A Life Apart. A Pilot Study of Residential Institutions for the Physically Handicapped and the Young Chronic Sick*. Tavistock Publications, London.

Moos, R. H., Gauvain, M., Lemke, S., Max, W. and Mehren, B. (1979). Assessing the social environments of sheltered care settings. *Gerontologist*, **19**, 74–82.

Neugarten, B. L., Havighurst, R. J. and Tobin, S. S. (1961). The measurement of life satisfaction. *Journal of Gerontology*, **16**, 134–143.

Norton, D., McLaren, R. and Exton-Smith, A. N. (1962). *An Investigation of Geriatric Nursing Problems in Hospital*. Churchill Livingstone, Edinburgh (reissued 1976).

Norwich, H. S. (1980). A study of nursing care in geriatric hospitals. *Nursing Times*, **76**, 292–295.

Office of Population Censuses and Surveys (1982). *General Household Survey 1980*. HMSO, London.

Office of Population Censuses and Surveys (1984). *Population Projections, 1981–2021*, Series PP2, No. 12. HMSO, London.

Parker, G. (1985). With Due Care and Attention. A Review of Research on Informal Care. Family Policy Studies Centre, London.

Pattie, A. H., Gilleard, C. J. and Bell, J. H. (1979). *The Relationship of the Intellectual and Behavioural Competence of the Elderly to their Present and Future Needs from the Community, Residential and Hospital Services*. Department of Clinical Psychology, Clifton Hospital, York.

Pembrey, S. (1980). *The Ward Sister — Key to Nursing; A Study of the Organisation of Individualized Nursing*. Royal College of Nursing, London.

Pincus, A. (1968). The definition and measurement of the institutional environment in homes for the aged. *Gerontologist*, **8**, 207–210.

Pincus, A. and Wood, V. (1970). Methodological issues in measuring the environment in institutions for the aged and its impact on residents. *Ageing and Human Development*, **1**, 117–126.

Plank, D. (1977). *Caring for the Elderly: Report of a Study of Various Means of Caring for Dependent Elderly People in Eight London Boroughs*. Greater London Council Research Memorandum, RM512, GLC, London.

Powell, C. and Crombie, A. (1974). The Kilsyth Questionnaire: a method of screening elderly people at home. *Age and Ageing*, **3**, 23–28.

Primrose, W. R. and Capewell, A. E. (1986). A survey of registered nursing homes in Edinburgh. *Journal of the Royal College of General Practitioners*, **36**, 125–128.

Rainey, C. G. E., Russel, W. F. and Silver, C. P. (1975). Long stay patients in the London Borough of Tower Hamlets. *Age and Ageing*, **4**, 247–254.

Raynes, N. B., Pratt, M. W. and Roses, S. (1979). *Organisational Structure and the Care of the Mentally Retarded*. Croom Helm, London.

Report of the Royal College of Physicians by the College Committee on Geriatrics (1981). Organic mental impairment in the elderly. Implications for research, education and the provision of services. *Journal of the Royal College of Physicians of London*, **15**, 141–167.

Revans, R. W. (1964). *Standards for Morale: Cause and Effect in Hospitals*. Oxford University Press for the Nuffield Provincial Hospital Trust, London.

Rhys-Hearn, C. (1979). Staffing geriatric wards: trials of a package. *Nursing Times* (Occasional Paper), **75** (11 and 12), 45–48, 52.

Rinke, C. L., Williams, J. J., Lloyds, K. and Scott, W. (1978). The effects of prompting and reinforcement on self-bathing by elderly residents in a nursing home. *Behaviour Therapy*, **9**, 873–881.

Robinson, R. A. (1971). Assessment scales in a psycho-geriatric unit, in G. Stocker *et al.* (Eds), *Assessment in Cerebrovascular Insufficiency*, Georg Thieme Verlag, Stuttgart.

Roe, P. and Guillem, V. (1978). The need for medical supervision in homes. *Health and Social Services Journal*, Feb. 10, 168–169.

Rosow, I. and Breslau, N. (1966). A Guttman health scale for the aged. *Journal of Gerontology*, **21**, 556–559.

Rowles, G. (1981). The surveillance zone as meaningful space for the aged. *The Gerontologist*, **21**, 304–311.

Rubin, S. G. and Davies, G. H. (1975). Bed blocking by elderly patients in general wards. *Age and Ageing*, **4**, 142–147.

Runciman, P. J. (1983). *Ward Sister at Work*. Churchill Livingstone, Edinburgh.

Runciman, W. G. (1966). *Relative Deprivation and Social Justice*. Routledge & Kegan Paul, London.

Sanford, J. R. A. (1975). Tolerance of debility in elderly dependants by supporters at home: its significance for hospital practice. *British Medical Journal*, **3**, 471–473.

Savage, B., Widdowson, T. and Wright, T. (1979). Improving the care of the elderly, in D. Towell and C. Harries (Eds), *Innovation in Patient Care: An Action Research Study of Change in a Psychiatric Hospital*. Croom Helm, London.

Senior, O. E. (1978). *Nurse/Patient Dependency*. Management Services, London.

Sinclair, I. (1971). *Hostels for Probationers*. Home Office Research Studies No. 6. HMSO, London.

Smith, R. G. and Lowther, C. P. (1976). Follow-up study of 200 admissions to a residential home. *Age and Ageing*, **5**, 176–180.

Stryker, R. (1981). *How to Reduce Employee Turnover in Nursing Homes and Other Health Care Organizations*. C. C. Thomas, Illinois.

Tarrier, N. and Larner, S. (1983). The effects of manipulation of social reinforcement on toilet requests on a geriatric ward. *Age and Ageing*, **12**, 234–239.

Thomson, D. (1983). Workhouse to nursing home: residential care of elderly people in England since 1840. *Ageing and Society*, **3**, 41–69.

Torrance, G. W. (1986). Measurement of health state utilities for economic appraisal: a review. *Journal of Health Economics*, **5**, 11–30.

Townsend, J. and Kimbell, A. (1975). Caring regimes in elderly persons' homes. *Health and Social Services Journal*, 11 October, 2286.

Townsend, P. (1957). *The Family Life of Old People*. Routledge & Kegan Paul, London.

Townsend, P. (1962). *The Last Refuge — A Survey of Residential Institutions and Homes for the Aged in England and Wales*. Routledge & Kegan Paul, London.

Townsend, P. (1965). On the likelihood of admission to an institution, in E. Shanas and G. F. Streib (Eds), *Social Structure and the Family Generational Relations*, pp. 163–187. Prentice-Hall, New York.

Townsend, P. (1973). The needs of the elderly and the planning of hospitals, in *Needs of the Elderly for Health and Welfare Services*, pp. 47–70. Institute of Biometry and Community Medicine, University of Exeter.

Townsend, P. (1979). Poverty in the United Kingdom: A Survey of Household Resources and Standards of living. Penguin, Harmondsworth.

Townsend, P. and Wedderburn, D. (1965). *The Aged in the Welfare State*, Occasional Papers on Social Administration, No. 14. Bell & Sons, London.

Twining, T. C. and Allen, D. G. (1981). Disability factors among residents of old people's homes. *Journal of Epidemiology and Community Health*, **35**, 205–207.

Wade, B., Sawyer, L. and Bell, J. (1983). *Dependency with Dignity*. Occasional Papers on Social Administration, No. 68. Bedford Square Press, London.

Walker, A. (1982). Dependency and old age. *Social Policy and Administration*, **16**, 115–135.

Wallis, D. and Cope, D. (1980). Pay-off conditions for organisational change in the hospital service, in K. D. Duncan, M. M. Gruneberg and D. Wallis (Eds), *Changes in Working Life*, pp. 459–480. John Wiley, London.

Warren, M. W. (1949). The role of a geriatric unit in a general hospital. *Ulster Medical Journal*, **18**, 3–12.

Wells, T. (1980). *Problems in Geriatric Nursing Care. A Study of Nurses' Problems in Care of Old People in Hospitals.* Churchill Livingstone, Edinburgh.

White, K. (1980). Nurse recruitment and retention in long-term care. *Journal of Long-Term Care Administrators*, **vii**, Fall, 25–36.

Whitehead, A. and Hunt, A. (1982). Elderly psychiatric patients: 5-year prospective study. *Psychological Medicine*, **12**, 149–157.

Wicks, M. and Rossiter, C. (1982). *Crises or Challenge? Family Care, Social Policy and Elderly People.* Study Commission on the Family, London.

Wilkin, D. (1986). *Theoretical and Conceptual Issues in the Measurement of Dependency.* Centre for Primary Care Research, University of Manchester.

Wilkin, D., Mashiah, T. and Jolley, D. J. (1978). Changes in behavioural characteristics of elderly populations of local authority homes and long-stay hospital wards, 1976–77. *British Medical Journal*, **2**, 1274–1276.

Willcocks, D., Peace, S. and Kellaher, L. (1987). *Private Lives in Public Places.* Tavistock Publications, London.

Williams, A. (1985). Economics of coronary artery by-pass grafting. *British Medical Journal*, **291**, 326–329.

Williamson, J. (1979). Notes on the historical development of geriatric medicine as a medical specialty. *Age and Ageing*, **8**, 144–148.

Williamson, J., Stokoe, I. H., Gray, S., Fisher, M., Smith, A., McGhee, A. and Stephenson, E. (1964). Old people at home: their unreported needs. *Lancet*, **i**, 1117–1120.

Wolfensberger, W. (1972). *Normalisation: One Principle of Normalisation in Human Services.* Leonard Crainford, Toronto.

Wright, K., (1985). Long-term care for the elderly: public versus private. *Public Money*, **5**, 52–54.

Research in the Nursing Care of Elderly People
Edited by P. Fielding
© 1987 John Wiley & Sons Ltd

CHAPTER 4

Evaluation of a Community-based Night Sitter Service

JANE DAWSON

Introduction

Last Scene of all,
That ends this strange eventful history,
Is second childishness, and mere oblivion,
Sans teeth, sans eyes, sans taste, sans everything.
(Jacques's Soliloquy on the Seven Ages of Man: Act II, Scene 7,
As You Like It, Shakespeare.)

One of the proudest claims of the United Kingdom has been that since the end of the Second World War the country's welfare state has been an example to the world. Unfortunately the economic recession of recent years has led to searching and sometimes acrimonious discussion as to how limited resources should be shared out amongst the various specialities and patient groups.

One such group, who by sheer weight of numbers cannot be ignored in resource allocation, are the dependent elderly. The establishment of a relief sitting service for psychogeriatric patients was the instigating factor in a study to examine the motivation and perceptions of the carers of such patients — the spouses or children who bore the brunt of the burden of caring for their severely dependent and confused relatives.

The sitting service was funded jointly by Hampshire Social Services and Southampton and South West Hants Health Authority. The service was managed by a paid co-ordinator who was an experienced psychiatric nurse. 'Sitters' were paid but untrained staff who went into the homes of psychogeriatric patients at regular intervals to care for them, relieving the caring relative for a few hours. The time and duration of this relief was entirely in response to relatives' wishes, and was arranged when the co-ordinator made her assessment visit. Thus some carers might receive three hours twice a week, others one day each week.

The sitting service was a new addition to a well-developed system of community care for the psychogeriatric patients in Southampton. Seventy-four admission and short-stay beds are used for planned short-stay relief admissions, and there is a fifteen place day hospital. There are 100 long-stay beds, and a relative support group is run weekly. In 1979 it was estimated that these facilities were serving a population of 50 000 people over 65 years of age. Four Community Psychogeriatric Nurses work with the Psychogeriatric Unit in Southampton. The philosophy of the whole psychogeriatric team, which embraces many different disciplines, is to provide the maximum possible community support for patients and their carers.

`It was the hope of the psychogeriatric team that the sitting service would provide a more appropriate form of care for those patients whose level of dependency was such that they required constant supervision. The confusional states of such patients is often worsened when they are removed, even to the protected environment of a day hospital, from their familiar surroundings. Nevertheless, regular relief to the caring relative was thought by the team to be essential if these patients were to continue to live at home.

The purposes of the research were two fold. Firstly to investigate what could broadly be termed motivation. how did carers come to assume and sustain their role as carers? What part did former role relationships play? Did social norms and expected behaviour influence the taking on of the caring role?

Secondly, to try to determine how the supportive services on which the philosophy of community care is based influenced the carers in the performance of their role as they saw it. Did these services sustain them in their role, or did they undermine or threaten it?

It seemed reasonable to assume that the carers' view of the support services would be largely dependent upon, and related to, the attitudes, values and assumptions which they brought to bear — even subconsciously — on their caring role.

It was issues such as these that the research was designed to address.

The Problem of Diagnosis and Identification

Precisely what physiological changes and clinically demonstrable signs and symptoms constitute a case for categorizing a person as a psychogeriatric patient?

Pitt (1974) gives the following definitions.

(A) *Mental illnesses*
   (i) *Organic*   1   Delerium (acute confusional state)
                       2   Dementia (chronic confusional state)
   (ii) *Functional*   1   Affective illness: depression, mania
                       2   Paranoid states
                       3   Neurosis
(B) *Personality and behaviour disorders*

However in the absence of definitive diagnostic techniques, the condition of being a psychogeriatric patient is far from clear-cut. Williams (1979) makes the point that physical illness in the elderly can produce symptoms similar to those listed above, and the difficulty of diagnosis is supported by others, notably Whitehead (1981). Bergmann (1978) suggests that failure to perform the limited role expected of him is the deciding factor by which an elderly person becomes a 'case'. Bergmann considers this limited role to be a negative one — not to create social or physical nuisance — and thus when an elderly person does so he or she becomes categorized as a psychogeriatric patient. Shepherd *et al.* (1966) could demonstrate no clear-cut distinction between 'cases' and 'normals' where neurosis was concerned, and Bergmann (1978) argues that this goes some way to explain what he terms the low social visibility of psychiatric disorders described by Simon (1966) and others.

The social and environmental factors which contribute to the diagnosis of psychogeriatric have been explained by several researchers. Hobman (1978) points out that the majority of people neither seek nor require help from medical and social agencies throughout the process of ageing. *Whitehead (1978)* reminds us how frequently the term senile is used as a term of abuse, and reiterates Hobman's (1978) point that old age does not inevitably produce mental decay. Whitehead (1978) also postulates the theory that the deterioration of memory, loss of emotional control, and inability to reason, which does occur in some elderly people is due to 'disuse' atrophy. By being forced by society into situations where they are not required or even permitted to think for themselves, Whitehead (1978) likens the elderly to institutional inmates. These people, he says, exhibit similar attitudes and signs of mental deterioration simply by disuse of such mental functions.

Along with the loss of a positive and satisfying role which Bergmann (1978) sees as crucial, Pitt (1974) lists other losses of a physical and emotional nature. Pitt (1974) cites status, income, health, company, familiar accommodation and the imminent threat of the loss of life itself. Pitt (1974) suggests, not unreasonably, that such losses contribute to psychiatric disorders, a view shared by Eisdorfer (1971).

Thus the diagnosis of an elderly person as a psychogeriatric is part medical and part socially determined, and its application may vary with the social context. Indeed several studies have shown that much psychiatric illness goes undiscovered and undiagnosed. Kay *et al.* (1964) showed that only about one-fifth of the elderly patients suffering from a psychiatric disorder were being cared for in hospital or local authority homes. Williamson *et al.* (1964) examined the physical and mental health of 200 people over 65 years of age and found 109 cases of psychiatric disorders previously undiagnosed. Perhaps these undiagnosed patients had not suffered the social crisis necessary to turn them into a 'case'.

As a consequence of this iceburg feature of psychogeriatric illness, the incidence in the population is based on studies which have specifically searched for such patients. Kay *et al.* (1964) in a sample of 297 people over 65 years of age found a prevalence rate of 10 per cent of people suffering from organic brain syndrome and 31 per cent with functional psychiatric disorders. Williamson *et al.* (1964) cite a prevalence of just over 25 per cent suffering from dementia in a study undertaken in Edinburgh. Parsons (1965) obtained a prevalence of 9.2 per cent of psychiatric conditions in a domiciliary sample, and using admission rates for a local psychiatric hospital concluded that for every elderly patient in hospital for a psychiatric condition there were 10 at home. This is half the rate identified by May *et al.* (1964) but Marsden (1978) agrees with Kay in estimating that about 10 per cent of those over 65 will show evidence of dementia. Adelstein (1968) demonstrated the steep rise in the inception of mental illness as age increases.

It is difficult to reconcile the differences in the estimation of psychogeriatric incidence, especially that of Williamson (1964). However, given that no definitive diagnostic tests exist for psychogeriatric conditions the subjective element in diagnosis could provide an explanation. The point is arguable.

The potential psychogeriatric population is demonstrably an area where further research is required. What is not in doubt is that overall the number of elderly suffering from such a condition will increase.

Clearly, medical and social provision will be considerably affected by the future demands of psychogeriatric patients and their carers of whom those in this study constitute a sample. The scale of such demands can be put in perspective by examining the proportion of the elderly to the total population.

The number of people in the United Kingdom over retirement age was 9.7 million in 1981, representing almost 18 per cent of the total population (OPCS, 1981). By 1991 the projected figure is 10.3 million, after which the numbers stabilize. More important than the overall rise of people over 65 is the rapid increase of the very elderly, and therefore those who are most frail and with highest dependency needs (see Table 1).

Table 1   Projected population over retirement age in Great Britain 1981 – 2001

Total numbers (millions)	1981	1991	2001
60/65 and over*	9.7	10.3	10.1
75 and over	4.1	3.1	3.8
85 and over	0.6	0.8	1.0
Rates of change	4.3	–2.0	–6.9
(% over decade)			
60/65 – 74			
75 – 84	24.1	16.6	1.1
85 and over	24.5	46.5	24.2

Source: *Census Guide One: Britain's elderly population* (OPCS, 1984).
* 60/65 and over means women aged 60 and over plus men aged 65 and over.

As Hunt (1978) observes, the possibility exists that those between 65 years and 75 years at the end of the century may be slightly healthier and better socially organized. Nevertheless, the probability is that the problems of housing, mobility, health and loneliness will be concentrated amongst particular groups. Hunt (1978) further showed that mobility and ability to perform personal care decreased as age increased. Caird and Gilmore (1976) looked at elderly people in three general practitioner groups, identifying factors which seemed to contribute to mental ill-health, in particular social isolation and lack of purpose. These findings in part support an Age Concern attitudinal study (1974) which showed disability as being highly correlated with loneliness, lack of significant others and dependence. Abrams (1977) surveyed 800 people over 75 years of age in four separate urban areas, 14 per cent of whom reported they suffered from depression.

Bearing in mind the theories of Pitt (1974), Eisdorfer (1977) and others that psychiatric disorders may in part be caused, or at least contributed to, by poor health and various social factors then a large group of elderly people are likely to be at risk.

In 1972 the DHSS (1972a) reported that since 1954 the proportion of patients over the age of 75 years in mental hospitals had doubled, whilst the number of hospital beds had been reduced by 30 per cent. By 1975 the DHSS (1975) stated that elderly people formed 20–25 per cent of the admissions to psychiatric hospitals. The 1976 DHSS document *Priorities for Health and Personal Social Services in England* estimated that about 2.5 per 1000 of the elderly people were in long-stay mental hospitals, and an even larger number with varying degrees of mental infirmity were living at home, or in some type of residential accommodation. The expenditure on services for them was £550 million in 1975/6, and the DHSS suggested a 3 per cent increase annually to 1980.

A Select Committee on Public Expenditure (1977) estimated that the peak in the elderly population by 1991 could require an increase in expenditure to meet medical and social needs of £300 million. Leaving aside the ethical and humanitarian issues, the only practical way of dealing with a problem of such magnitude is by increasing the range and extent of community care services. This is indeed recommended Government policy. *Better Services for the Mentally Ill* (DHSS, 1972a, p. 33) states:

> The aim always should be to respond to individual needs rather than to pursue generalised goals which for many of the mentally ill have little relevance . . . residential and day-care services should be conceived not as a self-contained system but as part of a broad range of options extending beyond the health and personal social services.

If services aimed at supporting the concept of community care are to be developed, then it is important to discover the impact such services have on the willingness of relatives to continue to care for their dependent relatives, and to understand how and why relatives assume a caring role.

Theoretical Perspectives

Reflecting the growing social concern over the problems of an ageing population has been the increase in research into various aspects of old age during the last twenty years. Robb (1967) instigated a public outcry with her work on the conditions in many geriatric wards and hospitals. It would not be an exaggeration to suggest that with the publication of Robb's work society at large was made vividly aware of the fact that dependency in old age was a major problem, and that positive steps would have to be taken to deal with it if the elderly infirm were to be treated in a humane and dignified manner. Following on from Robb's work, increasing public concern led to the DHSS publishing several reports and White Papers on care of the elderly (DHSS, 1972 a, b, 1975, 1976).

Further public criticism of conditions in geriatric and psychogeriatric wards led to the publication in 1972 of a DHSS Committee of Enquiry Report (DHSS, 1972b) and the care of the elderly mentally infirm was a major consideration in the DHSS (1975) document 'Better Services for the Mentally Ill'. This set out guidelines for the establishment of a more effective and sensitive service which would respond to this change. *Priorities for Health and Personal Social Services in England* (DHSS, 1976) emphasized the need to expand community services for the elderly, of whom those with mental infirmity formed a significant group.

One of the most surprising innovations to be suggested in recent years came in *A Happier Old Age* (DHSS, 1978). This was the proposed setting up of state-run nursing homes for the elderly mentally infirm. This suggestion was strongly attacked by MIND (1979) who saw this as a return to archaic practices of 'institutions' whose efficacy had already been disproved by Meacher (1972) and Thomas (1977). MIND set out their own extensive proposals for the care of the elderly mentally infirm, emphasizing again the need for expansion in community care facilities, and arguing the case against segregating such patients both from other elderly people and the wider society.

Whilst numerous studies have been concerned with the number and dependency of the elderly population, very little work has been carried out which provides the perspective of broader social theories. Thus the whole question of dependent elderly people is largely seen in purely pragmatic and piecemeal terms, rather than in a theoretical framework which might supply deeper understanding and a more comprehensive viewpoint.

To some extent the first steps towards the establishment of a more theoretical approach have come about through increased awareness of the effect on the family unit of having to care for a dependent elderly relative at home. Gilleard, Watt and Boyd (1981) and Levin (1982) have both discussed the problems facing the supporters of the elderly mentally infirm in the community, but rather surprisingly most of the work in this area has been carried out at the behest of the Equal Opportunities Commission. In 1980 the Commission (EOC, 1980) reported on a survey into the implications for women of community care policies. The impetus behind the Commission's interest was their contention, supported by Townsend (1957), Cartwright, Hockey and Anderson (1973) and their own 1978 survey that the great majority of carers for handicapped and dependent elderly people were women. The Commission took the view that the concept of community care — which is the cornerstone of recent social policy – discriminates against women on two counts. Firstly, that the community care philosophy (i.e. care by women) is based on the erroneous assumption that married women do not take paid employment, and secondly, that because of this assumption, many female carers are excluded from, or find it difficult to obtain, financial support in their caring task. The Commission further suggests that because of this exploitation of women as cheap labour, the option of community care is attractive to Government because it costs less. Emotional costs to carers brought about by the stress inherent in their caring role is ignored when social policy is determined.

The cost, both in emotional and financial terms has been examined also by Nissel and Bonnerjea (1981, 1982) who broadly support the EOC's viewpoint.

Moroney (1976) looked at community care from a different perspective. In an analysis of social policies directed at two specific client groups, the mentally handicapped and the elderly, Moroney examined the extent to which measures which purport to encourage community care do in fact achieve this objective. He pointed out that resource allocation has not kept pace with the increasing number of people for whom community care is the chosen option, which in any case, says Moroney, is an illusory concept if the choice is between concerned care at home and residential care of poor quality.

On the other hand, the paucity of resources for community care has resulted in services being withheld where family support is presumed to exist. Instead of helping families to care for their mentally handicapped or elderly relative, policies may actually cause breakdown and subsequent institutionalization when families decide they can no longer carry on. Moroney (1976) therefore argues that the relationship between statutory and family support (ideologically the State *vis-à-vis* private), is not complementary, but an either/or dichotomy.

Feminist writers such as Taylor (1979) and Ungerson (1982) have begun to question the role of women in caring for dependent relatives. Johnson (1975) points out that the whole philosophy of families caring for their elderly dependents is based on an erroneous understanding of 'the family' as a term which always implies a social unit of known dimensions and inherent resources and that this is demonstrably not the case (Bott, 1971). Johnson (1975) suggests society has excluded the elderly from the process of social exchange and a reciprocal gift relationship by basing response to need on a system which turns the elderly into passive recipients who are thus made more dependent.

Williams (1979) makes the point that quality of life is always subjective, and that services provided should be related to how elderly people themselves view their needs. Professionals are seen by Williams as bringing predominantly middle-class attitudes to a situation and therefore offer 'solutions' which are unrealistic for a large section of their elderly clients.

One of the aims of this study was to see how services were perceived by, and influential upon, caring relatives. Williams's argument provides the basis of a hypothesis which encapsulates that aim, and which was examined in the study: *Community services to psychogeriatric patients may exert both negative and positive influences on caring relatives in the performance of their role.*

Although the theories discussed above provide an alternative interpretation of support services, they do not offer an explanatory theory of the nature of the relationship between services provided and carers' motivation, or of the mechanisms at work to sustain the carers' motivation.

Ungerson (1982) touches upon motivation when she maintains that caring for is viewed as evidence of 'caring about'. The Equal Opportunities Commission report (1980) does set down the carer's expressed viewpoint through verbatim quotes and in *Who Cares for the Carers?* (EOC, 1982b) states '. . . there is no doubt that for many people the emotional rewards of caring far outweigh the disadvantages . . .' However, work on carers of sick or handicapped children does provide some fruitful ideas.

Davis (1963) suggests that guilt was a central feature to the parents of children who had contracted polio, and that they accommodated their situation by staging a public performance of a well adjusted family unit. Voysey (1975) supports the theory of a performance with regard to parents of mentally handicapped children, but argues that this performance is modelled on the theories presented to them by visiting agencies. Voysey defines four theoretical dimensions as crucial: religion, medical science, psychiatry and sociology. Voysey's construct of legitim- izing theories is supported in part by the work of Chodoff (1964), Burton (1974) and Wilkins (1979).

Given that agencies officially charged with the care and control of elderly people exist, then the possibility of some modelling of behaviour in caring relatives of psychogeriatric patients cannot be dismissed.

Regardless of the influence of controlling agencies, participants in a relationship, whether parents, spouses or children do have beliefs about how they should behave — norms governing conduct. Birenbaum (1976) defines norms as socially expected and accepted forms of behav- iour, able to be sustained and altered as occasion demands. The norms implicit in a social relationship thus constitute the script for the perform- ance of that role.

Turner (1962) argues that modification of role-performance takes place, role-making as well as role-taking. If official agencies influence carers as Voysey suggests, then clearly the carer's role is to some extent 'made' by them.

Goffman (1969) points out that when an individual stages a perform- ance it is implicit that others take the performance seriously. But, Goffman asks, does the performer himself believe in his performance? In this context, to what extent and by what means have carers come to internalize the caring role which they perform?

The vital importance of research in the formulation of social policy concerned with the elderly in the community was the central theme of a seminar sponsored by the DHSS in September 1982 (*DHSS, 1983*). The effect on carers of the various support services was a point referred to by many of the speakers, together with the assumptions behind such services. This study was executed in an effort to discover a little more about the burden of dependency from the point of view of those who carry it, namely the carers.

Methodology

The paucity of work in this field virtually dictated the need to adopt a grounded theory approach. Thus a self-completion questionnaire or structured interviews with carers was inappropriate. Pilot interviews with carers had highlighted the centrality of the concepts of duty and self-esteem. If these concepts were to be explored in order to elicit commonly held themes, then the required sample would be too large for observation methods, given the constraints of time and practicality.

The methodology finally adopted was twofold. Firstly an assessment document (see Table 2), and secondly tape-recorded focused interviews with carers. In addition to demographic information on the patient, the carer, and other members of the household, the assessment document measured the dependence of the patient in activities of daily living such as washing, dressing, feeding, and incontinence. A fairly basic measure of mental state was also included (see Table 3).

Such an assessment document would provide a background and context to the study. Of equal importance, the comparability or differences of patients and carers could be evaluated, and related to the interview data. This assessment document was based on work carried out in Southampton on assessment of physical handicap (Cantrell, Dawson and Glastonbury, 1983) and on Wade and Sawyer's (1983)

Table 2   Structure of household

Carers code	Sex of carer	Age of carer	Relationship of carer to dependent relative	Others in household	Age of dependent relative	Sex
A	M	74	Husband	Nil	77	F
B	F	71	Wife	Nil	77	M
C	F	75	Wife	Nil	81	M
D	M	71	Husband	Nil	74	F
E	M	83	Husband	Nil	83	F
F	F	75	Wife	Nil	76	M
G	M	76	Husband	Nil	77	F
H	M	67	Husband	Nil	65	F
I/C	M	56	Son	Daughter-in-law	96	F
J/C	F	44	Daughter	Nil	76	M
K/C	F	53	Daughter	Grandson	86	F
L/C	F	26	Daughter	Wife	68	M
M/C	F	67	Daughter	Nil	88	F
N/C	F	64	Daughter	Nil	87	F
O/C	F	48	Daughter	Son-in-law	76	F
P	F	81	Wife	Nil	84	M
Q	F	79	Wife	Nil	84	M
R	F	66	Wife	Nil	71	M
S	M	77	Husband	Daughter	82	F
T	F	72	Wife	Daughter	74	M

Table 3   Dependency of psychogeriatric patient

Carers code	Length of care	Mobility Code Able to walk	Unable to walk	Incontinence Urine	Faeces	Feeding code	Mental State (coded)
A	4	1	—	1	1	1	39
B	4	1	—	2	2	2	48
C	4	1	—	2	1	1	49
D	3	3	—	1	1	2	47
E	4	1	—	3	1	1	51
F	4	1	—	4	2	2	55
G	3	1	—	1	1	1	41
H	4	1	—	3	2	1	45
I/C	4	1	—	1	1	1	40
J/C	4	1	—	2	2	1	51
K/C	2	1	—	1	1	1	36
L/C	4	3	—	1	1	2	55
M/C	3	1	—	2	1	3	46
N/C	4	1	—	2	1	1	48
O/C	2	1	—	1	1	1	41
P	3	2	—	2	2	1	38
Q	2	1	—	1	1	2	39
R	1	1	—	1	1	1	44
S	5	3	—	3	3	3	46
T	4	3	—	3	1	1	43

Key to coding
Length of care

3–6 months	1
6 months – 1 year	2
1 year – 2 years	3
1 year – 5 years	4
5 years +	5

Feeding

Feeds self	1
Needs watching	2
Requires feeding	3

Urinary continence

Is never incontinent	1
Is sometimes incontinent	2
Is always incontinent	3
Has a catheter/appliance	4

Faecal continence

Is never incontinent	1
Is sometimes incontinent	2
Is always incontinent	3

Able to Walk

Able to walk unaided	1
Able to walk with Zimmer/stick	2
Able to walk only with assistance	3

Mental state assessment
Mental state assessed from 24 items, scored 1–3.
Aggregate minimum score 24 (least mental deterioration).
Aggregate maximum score 72 (24 × 3) (severe mental deterioration).

assessment of elderly people. The document was constructed by the researcher but completed by the co-ordinator of the scheme following referral of a patient for a sitter.

The focused interviews took place in the patient and carer's home. They were conducted a few weeks after carers first received a sitter, an appointment convenient to the carer having been made by the researcher in person. The use of a tape-recorder was very well accepted, in fact it enabled the interview to be conducted more in the nature of a conversation, which undoubtedly increased the freedom with which carers responded.

The service came into operation in January 1983, and efforts were made to interview all 30 carers who received a sitter during the period from January 1983 to July 1983.

From these 30, two were interviewed as part of the pilot study, giving a sample of 28 for the actual study. Of those, two patients died and one was admitted to hospital before the interview could be conducted. Two carers changed their minds about having a sitter, and one was excluded from the sample on the grounds of age as the patient was only 60. Another case was excluded as the main carers were non-resident children, the sitter being provided to support a married couple who were both mentally confused. No carer refused to be interviewed, though one interview with a caring son was not carried out as he failed to keep the appointment, and subsequent efforts to contact him failed. Non-response thus totalled eight cases, leaving a possible 20 cases in the sample.

By the end of July 1983, thirteen caring spouses had been interviewed. Interviews were becoming repetitive in that each new carer interviewed was responding in a manner which echoed, on occasions almost verbatim, the respondents of previous interviews. Themes which seemed to be central to carers had emerged from early interviews, and later respondents were reiterating these themes, rather than raising new ones. At this point, only three children caring for dependent parents had been interviewed during the initial six months. It therefore seemed more fruitful to interview a larger sample of caring children. As the relationship with the dependent patient was fundamentally different, it seemed highly likely that data from this source would provide either different themes, or an alternative perspective on them, from those of caring spouses. For this reason only caring children who received the service were included in the study from August to November 1983. Four referrals were for caring children in this period, and all were interviewed.

A total of 20 interviews were conducted, lasting from 45 minutes to two hours. The profile (Tables 2 and 3) shows that thirteen respondents were caring for spouses and seven for parents. Of the spouses six were husbands caring for wives, and seven were wives caring for husbands. Only one son caring for a parent was interviewed, the remaining six caring children were daughters.

The Motivation of Carers, and Their Perceptions of Support Services

Patient Dependency

Analysis of the assessment document while not specifically bearing upon the theoretical aspects of the study does serve to illustrate the level of dependency and to provide relevant background information for the analysis of other issues.

Tables 2 and 3 give a profile of the patients and their carers. Fourteen households (70 per cent) consisted solely of patient and carer. Two caring spouses (S and T) had children still living at home. In one of these the couple's daughter was mentally handicapped, in the other their daughter worked full-time. One caring daughter (L/C) looked after both parents as her mother was in poor physical health, and another (K/C) had her own 23-year-old son (the patient's grandson) living in the household. Two caring children (I/C and O/C) were married and had taken their parent into their own marital home.

The mean age of patients was 79 years, the youngest being 65 years and the oldest 96.

Mental state of patients was assessed by encoding the frequency with which 24 separate behaviour patterns occurred on a three-point scale. Thus a patient who was never noisy at night scored 1, occasionally noisy scored 2, always noisy at night scored 3. These scores were then added to give a total score. The lowest achievable score was therefore 24, the highest 72. From this scale thirteen patients were classified as moderate dementia and seven as severe.

Analysis of Interview Data

The data from the interviews was first analysed to examine whether Voysey's four dimensions of legitimizing theories — religion, medical science, psychiatry and sociology — were valid.

The age of most of the caring spouses had led the researcher to the expectation that considerable use would be made of religion. This did not prove to be the case. None regarded the illness as an act of God, retribution or a cross to be borne. However, four spouses (less than 25 per cent) did claim that their ability to continue with the task was strengthened by their religious faith.

Only one of the children caring for a parent regarded religion as a help in coping with her task, but in a manner different to that of the spouses quoted. For Mrs O/C the spiritual closeness she felt for her dead father was both a reason for caring for her mother and a way of coping with the burden of care.

One son who described himself as a lay-priest, and could therefore have been expected to have an approach to life based on religious faith did not use religion as a model for his actions as a carer, but regarded the task as the 'natural' thing to do. Religion was not then a legitimizing factor for these carers.

Carers in the study also differed in their use of the medical model. They did not seek for explanation of the illness as a fault of physiological mechanisms which would be corrected if rigorous treatment or drug regimes were followed, as did the parents of handicapped children. This may be due in part to the fact that all but two of the dependent patients in the sample were of an age whereby, even if they were not suffering from a psychogeriatric condition they would be nearing the end of their expected life-span. The need to seek a cure is arguably much less pressing, or relevant. Certainly carers in the sample seemed to regard as inevitable the progressive and intractable nature of the illness.

Whilst rejecting the use of a medical model in seeking a cause or dictating a life-style (i.e. centred around treatment), some carers did make use of this model to cast the dependent relative in the sick role, using this as an explanation of trying and bizarre behaviour. All spouses used the model in this way, and to justify their acceptance of services. Caring children made very little use of a medical model.

The nature of psychogeriatric conditions and the familial relationship of the carers to the dependants virtually precludes the application of the other two models to the study. There is only one illustration in the data of a social or psychological factor being seen as causing the illness. One spouse indicated that the marital relationship had never been a very happy one, and made it clear that she regarded her past actions in doing everything for her husband was partly responsible for his condition.

The carers then did not use the legitimating theories explored as a central focus. There was no evidence that they needed to find such a construct to help them make sense of the illness. This difference in attitude can best be understood in terms of the varying nature of the expected norms within the carer/dependant relationship in the sample with those of parent/dependent child.

Pilot interviews had indicated that the concept of duty played a major part in the acceptance of the caring role. This was borne out by the subsequent research, as without exception all carers referred to their caring role as a duty. Furthermore, this sense of duty was bound up with feelings of extreme guilt with regard to utilization by some carers of support facilities.

The concept of duty appears to be absolutely pivotal to all carers' attitudes to their role, but meant significantly different things to caring children than it did to caring spouses.

For caring children duty was reciprocity for their own past dependence, and affection for their parent. 'Caring for' was 'caring about', and any other course was unthinkable. Because of this meaning of duty to them the concept of guilt at accepting support services was minimal to caring children. They viewed such services as a practical way of coping with their task.

This was in marked contrast to the attitude of spouses. For them duty was dictated by — indeed virtually synonymous with — their marital role. These carers saw the marital role as supplying the norms by which their assumption and continuation of the caring role came about. Herein lies the key to the relationship between duty and guilt. Utilizing services which relieved them of some of the burden by removing the dependent spouse from the home caused them to experience overwhelming guilt at abdicating from their marital role. Their guilt was such that short-stay and day placement was refused time and again, even when the caring spouse was on the verge of physical and emotional collapse.

The data indicates then that there is an optimum point at which services are no longer perceived by caring spouses as supporting the caring role but of removing it altogether, thus inducing severe role-conflict.

For caring children support services cause no role-conflict in sustaining a role which, while important, is not dominant. Because they are part of other role-sets also, the caring role is not threatened when relieved.

Spouses on the other hand, see their role as husband and wife as being constituted by norms which demand that they and they alone should do the caring. Marriage is after all an exclusive relationship.

Anything less, any diminution of the caring role threatens their self-esteem as responsible husband or wife fulfilling their role obligations, and may cast doubt on the validity of their marital role, which at their age and situation in life constitutes the only significant role they retain.

Conclusion and Implications

The hypothesis which the study set out to examine, that is that community services have both negative and positive influences in the performance of the caring role was supported. The manner in which these influences operate can be explained by an understanding of the degree to which the caring role fulfils the needs of the self for the carer.

Relatives, whether spouses or children, take on and continue the caring role because in doing so they fulfil their role *vis-à-vis* the dependent patient. The reciprocity of the caring role which enables them to continue caring lies in the maintenance of their self-esteem, and their confirmation of the validity of their past role relationship with the patient. The conception carers have of their role influences the way in which services are viewed. Those for whom the caring role is of major importance regard services which appear to take over the care (such as short-stay and day care) as excluding them from such a role. Carers for whom this role is one of a set of roles are likely to regard all support services as helpful and supporting in its execution.

The sitting service, being provided in the home and entirely at the time requested by the caring relative, posed no such threat. They were still in control of the caring situation as the sitter was under their direction, and in their environment. No role-conflict was evoked, so feelings of guilt were not aroused.

One of the concerns of policy-makers is that the rise in the number of dependent elderly people will not be matched by an equal number of children willing to care for them. This study indicates that it will, and they will expect to make use of a variety of support services. The question of whether spouses will hold similar views on their caring role is more problematic. If the caring role is an integral part of the marital role, then will subsequent generations who may have contracted two or three marriages during their lifetime hold the view that caring for their dependent partner is their exclusive role? And will children who 'acquire' a step-parent in their adulthood have the same sense of duty towards them as to a natural parent?

Whilst these questions must be left for future research, one of the immediate conclusions is that caring relatives require the availability of a range of support services, from which those most appropriate at a particular point in time can be offered. For some carers, particularly spouses, day-care or short-stay admission was too big a jump from the total care they themselves had been giving. The acceptance of the sitting service perhaps indicates that if this were the first step in the acceptance of help, carers would be able to make use of more complete care for their dependent relative as the condition progressed. In this way carers might be more willing to accept external help, free from guilt, before the point was reached at which they themselves became physically and mentally exhausted, and unable to continue their caring role.

References

Abrams M. (1977). *Beyond Three Score Years and Ten*. Age Concern, London.
Adelstein, A. M. (1968). The epidemiology of mental illness in an English city. *Social Psychiatry*, **3**, 47–59.
Age Concern (1974). *The Attitudes of the Retired and Elderly*. Age Concern, London.
Bergmann, K. (1978). *The Aged: Their Understanding and Care*. Wolfe Publishing, London.
Birenbaum, A. (1976). *Norms, Rules and Deviance*. Praeger, New York.
Bott, E. (1957). *Family and Social Network*. Tavistock Institute of Human Relations, London.
Burton, L. (1974). *Care of the Child Facing Death*. Routledge & Kegan Paul, London and Boston.
Caird, F. I. and Gilmore, A. J. J. (1976). Domiciliary health and welfare services for the elderly in Glasgow: use and needs. *Community Health*, 7, 128–134.
Cantrell, E., Dawson, J. and Glastonbury, G. (1983). *Prisoners of Handicap*. University of Southampton.
Cartwright, A., Hockey, L. and Anderson, J. (1973). *Life Before Death*. Routledge & Kegan Paul, London and Boston.
Chodoff, P. (1963). Stress, defences and coping behaviour: Observations in parents of children with malignant disease. *American Journal of Psychiatry*, **120**, 743–749.
Davis, F. (1963). *Passage Through Crisis*. Bobbs-Merrill, Indianapolis.
Department of Health and Social Security (1972a). *Better Services for the Mentally Ill*. HMSO, London.
Department of Health and Social Security (1972b). *Whittingham Hospital: Report of the Committee of Enquiry*. HMSO, London.
Department of Health and Social Security (1975). *The Way Forward: Priorities in Health and Social Services*. HMSO, London.
Department of Health and Social Security (1976). *Priorities for Health and Personal Social Services in England*. HMSO, London.
Department of Health and Social Security (1978). *A Happier Old Age*. HMSO, London.

Department of Health and Social Security (1981a). *Report of Study in Community Care*. HMSO, London.
Department of Health and Social Security (1983). *Research contributions to the development of social policy*: essays based on the seminar 'Support for elderly people living in the community', sponsored by DHSS and held at the University of East Anglia, September 1982. HMSO, London.
Eisdorfer, C. (1977). *Cognitive and Emotional Disturbance in the Elderly: Clinical Issue Note*. Paper presented to a Symposium and Workshop, Jerusalem.
Equal Opportunities Commission (1980). *The Experience of Caring for Elderly and Handicapped Dependants*. EOC, Manchester.
Equal Opportunities Commission (1981). *Behind Closed Doors*. EOC, Manchester.
Equal Opportunities Commission (1982a). *Caring for the Elderly and Handicapped*. EOC, Manchester.
Equal Opportunities Commission (1982b). *Who Cares for the Carers: Opportunities for those caring for the Elderly and Handicapped*. EOC, Manchester.
Gilleard, C. J., Watt, G. and Boyd, W. D. (1981). *Problems in Caring for the Elderly Mentally Infirm at Home*. International Congress of Gerentology.
Goffman, E. (1969). *Presentation of Self in Everyday Life*. Allen Lane, London.
Hobman, D. (1978). *The Social Challenge of Ageing*. Croom Helm, London.
Hunt, A. (1978). *The Elderly at Home*. For Office of Population and Census Statistics, HMSO, London.
Johnson, M. (1975). Old age and the gift relationship. *New Society*, **31**, No. 649.
Kay, D. W., Beamish, P. and Roth, M. (1964). Old age mental disorders in Newcastle upon Tyne. *British Journal of Psychiatry*, **110**, 146–158.
Levin, E. (1982). *The Supporters of Confused Elderly Persons in the Community*. National Institute of Social Work, London.
Marsden, C. D. (1978). The diagnosis of dementia, in A. Isaacs and F. Post (Eds), *Studies in Geriatric Psychiatry*. John Wiley & Sons, London.
Meacher, M. (1972). *Taken for a Ride*. Longman, Harlow.
MIND (1979). *Mental Health of Elderly: MINDS Response to DHSS. Discussion paper 'A Happer Old Age'*. MIND: London.
Moroney, R. (1976). *Family and the State. Considerations for Social Policy*. Longman.
Nissel, M. and Bonnerjea, L. (1982). *Family Care of the Elderly Handicapped: Who Pays?* Policy Studies Institute, London.
Office of Population and Census Statistics (1981). *Demographic Review*. HMSO, London.
Office of Population and Census (1984). *Census Guide One: Britain's Elderly Population*. See Table 1 source.
Parsons, P. L. (1965). Mental health of Swansea's old folk. *British Journal of Preventive and Social Medicine*, **19**, 43–47.
Pitt, B. (1974). *Psychogeriatrics. An Introduction to the Psychiatry of Old Age*. Churchill Livingstone, London and Edinburgh.
Robb, B. (1967). *Sans Everything*. Thomas Nelson, London.
Select Committee on Public Expenditure Session 1976–77. Chapter V, *Spending on the Health and Personal Social Services*. HMSO, London.

Shepherd, M., Cooper, B., Brown, A. and Kalton, G. W. (1966). *Psychiatric Illness in General Practice*. University Press London, Oxford.

Simon, A. (1966). Mental health of community resident versus hospitalised aged, in Simon, A. and Epstein, L. J. (Eds), *Ageing in Modern Society*, pp. 161–169. American Psychiatric Association, Washington.

Taylor, J. (1979). Hidden labour and the National Health Service, in P. Atkinson, *Prospects for the National Health*. Croom Helm, London.

Thomas, P. (1977). Experiences of two preventive clinics for the elderly. *British Medical Journal*, **2**, pp. 164–166.

Townsend, P. (1957). *The Family Life of Old People*. Penguin, Harmondsworth.

Turner, T. (1962). Role-taking: process versus conformity, in A. Rose, *Human Behaviour and Social Processes*. Routledge & Kegan Paul, London.

Ungerson, C. (1981). *Women, Work and the Caring Capacity of the Community*. Report for Social Services Research Council.

Ungerson, C. (1982). *Women and Caring. Skills, Tasks and Taboos*. Paper to British Sociological Association Conference on Gender in Society Manchester.

Voysey, M. (1975). *A Constant Burden*. Routledge & Kegan Paul, London and Boston.

Wade, B. and Sawyer, L. (1983). *Dependency with Dignity. Different Provision for the Elderly*. National Council of Voluntary Organization Publication.

Whitehead, T. (1978). *In the Service of Old Age: the Welfare of Psychogeriatric Patients*. Harmondsworth, London.

Whitehead, T. (1981). Care of the elderly mentally ill in impending old age, in R. Shegog (Ed.), *The Impending Crisis of Old Age*. Oxford University Press, Oxford.

Wilkins, D. (1979). *Caring for the Mentally Handicapped Child*. Croom Helm, London.

Williams, I. (1979). *The Care of the Elderly in the Community*. Croom Helm, London.

Williamson, J. (1964). Old people at home: their unreported needs. *The Lancet*, 23–25.

Research in the Nursing Care of Elderly People
Edited by P. Fielding
© 1987 John Wiley & Sons Ltd

CHAPTER 5

A Clinical Trial of Incontinence Garments

MANDY FADER

Introduction

Urinary incontinence is a common and disabling problem. Much has been written about the embarrassment, discomfort, odour and skin problems that sufferers may experience, and of the drain on nursing time and resources that it causes (see for example, Norton, 1982; Norton, McLaren and Exton-Smith, 1975).

Despite the development of new ways of treating urinary incontinence, investigation and treatment are not appropriate or available for all sufferers and many must manage their problem with incontinence aids. There is a vast range of aids to choose from, but few are fully effective. Apart from incontinence garments, no satisfactory aid has been devised for women. Although men have a greater choice, with male appliances and sheath drainage systems as alternatives to incontinence garments, these have their limitations and may be unsatisfactory for men with a retracted penis or those who have difficulty in applying them. Consequently, a large proportion of incontinent people manage their problem with incontinence garments.

A postal survey by Thomas *et al.* (1980) found that in the under 65 years age group 8.5 per cent of women and 1.6 per cent of men admit to urinary incontinence twice or more a month. This figure rises to 11.6 per cent of women and 6.9 per cent of men in the over 65 years age group. It is interesting to note that when validating the questionnaire used in the survey by interviewing 178 of those admitting incontinence 24 (71 per cent) of the 34 with moderate or severe incontinence were receiving no incontinence aids or other help from the health or social services. In fact prevalence estimates made by the Health and Social Services for the same study showed that only 0.2 per cent of women and 0.1 per cent of men aged 15–65 and 2.5 per cent of women and 1.3 per cent of men aged 65 and over were known to be incontinent. In institutions, especially for the elderly, the figures are higher although reports vary widely. Milne (1976) gave a prevalence of urinary incontinence amongst older patients in hospital as 13–48 per cent. In residential homes for the elderly 17 per cent are reported to be incontinent of urine (Masterton *et al.*, 1980). With an estimated 200 000 beds in geriatric, psychogeriatric and Part III homes in the UK, it would be expected that from 25 000 to 85 000 of the occupants may suffer with urinary incontinence.

✶ In this chapter I describe a trial of incontinence garments which was funded by the DHSS and published in full as Health Equipment Information No. 159 (Fader *et al.*, 1986). An incontinence garment consists of an absorbent pad held against the body to absorb urine. Special pants may be used or the absorbent may be fashioned into a garment (Figures 1–7).

All pads have an absorbent core which is generally made of fluffed wood pulp or wadding. Both these consist of cellulose fibres extracted from trees, the fibres being formed into sheets of tissue paper to make up cellulose wadding. Some products contain a super-absorbency gel to increase the absorbency. The absorbent is held in place by a 'coverstock', which comes into contact with the skin. This is a non-woven material and may be made from viscose, polyester, polyethylene or polypropylene.

Most pads have a waterproof backing which is almost universally made from fine gauge polyethylene film. Most films are micro-embossed to reduce the contact of the polyethylene with the skin.

Special pants may be used to hold the pad in place. A variety of methods for securing the pad to the pants are used, such as a pocket or pouch, but some pants are designed to be particularly close fitting so that these are not necessary. Pants are available with a waterproof gusset which are designed to be used with pads which have no polyethylene backing. Most pants are 'pull-on' in style, but several are made to be either front or side opening supposedly to ease application of the pad or the pants.

As incontinent garments are not prescribable under the Drug Tariff provisions it is up to each health district to provide a range of incontinent garments, usually made available through the community nursing services. However, the cost of providing incontinence garments is very

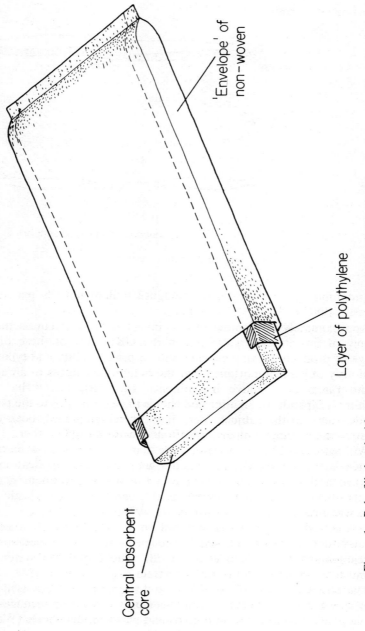

'Envelope' of non-woven

Layer of polythylene

Central absorbent core

Figure 1 Pulp filled pad with non-woven coverstock and polyethylene backing (pad may be shaped)

Fine, elasticated mesh

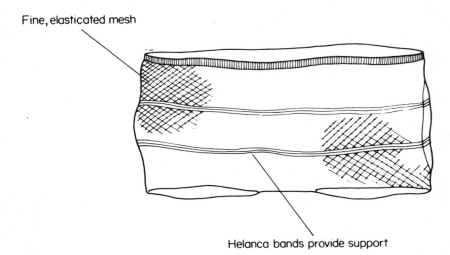

Helanca bands provide support

Figure 2   Stretch pants

considerable, a recent estimate being 12 million pounds per annum (HSSC, 1984).

Approximately 26 companies are involved in the manufacture or supply of incontinence garments in the UK. Most of these offer a range of products varying considerably in price, quality and type. It is obviously of great importance that the patient has access to an appropriate range of effective incontinence garments, but it has been extremely difficult for an informed choice to be made due to the paucity of literature on the subject. Very few clinical trials have been done, most of them being comparisons of one garment with another.

Willington (1969) first described the marsupial pants, now marketed as 'Kanga Pants'. He demonstrated a greater ease in application, less leakage and a saving in nursing time when 80 incontinent geriatric inpatients started using Kanga Pants and pads instead of plastic pants with wadding inserts (Willington *et al.*, 1972).

The Kanga system was compared with the Molnlycke Maxi-Plus Diapers and stretch pants when used by fifteen female patients in a psychogeriatric unit (Tam *et al.*, 1978). The Molnlycke system was found to be superior to the Kanga system.

The Molnlycke Maxi-Plus Diapers and stretch pants were used by 54 long-stay geriatric patients who had been previously been managed with tissue paper incontinence underpads and plastic under sheets (Watson,

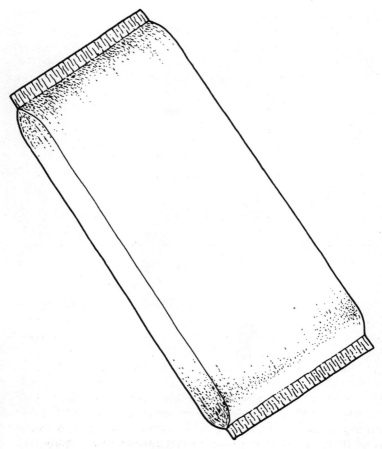

Figure 3 Pulp filled single pad with non-woven coverstock and no backing

1980). A 90 per cent saving in incontinence pads and a 50 per cent
saving in laundry costs was made using the Molnlycke system.

Sheperd and Blanin (1980) compared the Kanga system, the
Molnlycke system and Sandra plastic pants with wadding inserts. These
were used by 20 incontinent out-patients and the Kanga system was
found to be superior. It was stressed that no single system suited
everyone and that individual needs varied and should be provided for.
The authors also emphasized that only a small population sample was
used.

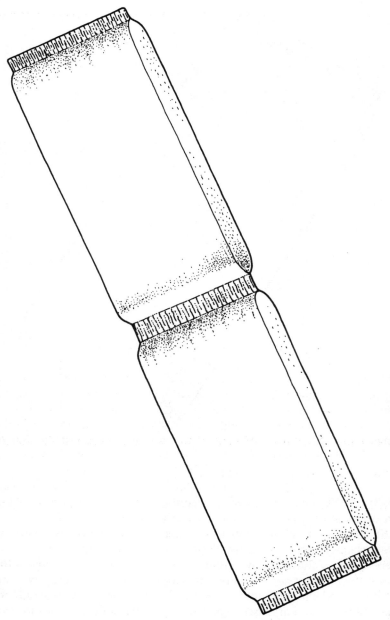

Figure 4   Pulp filled double pad with non-woven coverstock and no backing

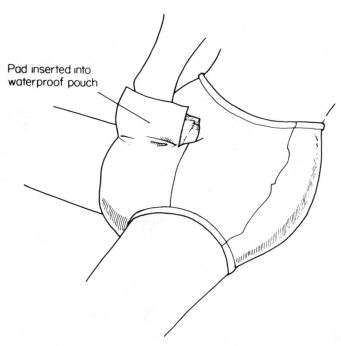

Pad inserted into
waterproof pouch

Figure 5   Pants with waterproof pouch (marsupial)

The Kanga system was compared with the Sandra plastic pants containing the Smith and Nephew Bambi pads by Bainton, Blanin and Shepherd (1982). Fifty-one female patients living at home took part in the crossover trial. Ninety-eight per cent of the patients preferred the Kanga pants. Sixty-five per cent of the patients preferred the Bambi pad and the Kanga pad was criticized for being too bulky. Both systems kept a similar proportion of patients dry during the day and night.

Malone-Lee, McCreery and Exton-Smith (1982) assessed the acceptability of eight incontinence garments for 113 patients living in Part III accommodation and in their own homes. The study showed that the needs of the patients in Part III were very different to those in the community. The Molnlycke T Form pad or Maxi-Plus pad and stretch pants most suited the subjects in Part III. Patients living in the community needed to be offered a range of garments. This would be met by the Kanga Standard or Kanga Lady pants with the Standard or single pad, the Smith and Nephew Dandeliners and the Molnlycke Maxi-Plus pad and T Form pad with stretch pants. It was emphasized

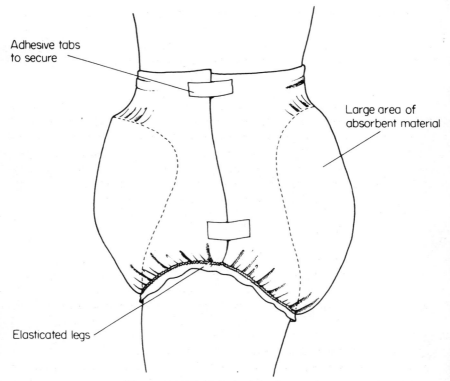

Figure 6   All-in-one adult diaper

that manufacturers should pay particular attention to the aesthetic qualities of the products. The authors also highlighted the need for more
information about the structure and constituents of incontinence
garments to be made available to those involved in their purchase.

In addition to these clinical trials a number of articles have been
written in the nursing press giving opinions with limited clinical trials
on various newly introduced products (see for example, Schofield and
Schofield, 1981).

However, with the large and increasing number of incontinence
garments available it is not yet possible to know which would be most
suitable for a wide range of different needs, for patients in hospital, in
Part III accommodation and in the community.

The clinical trials to date involved trying incontinence garments on
a sample of patients without consideration being given as to the suit-
ability of the garment for the patient. Incontinence garments vary

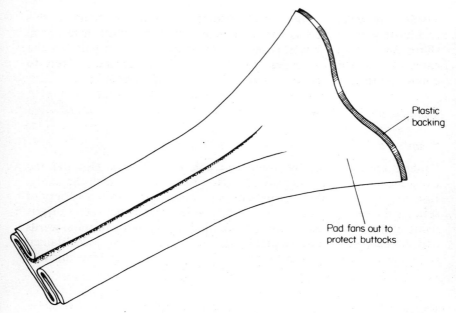

Plastic
backing

Pad fans out to
protect buttocks

Figure 7   Wing-folded pad

considerably in size and type to suit different patients with different severities of incontinence. Assessment of products by one group of patients alone obviously limits the value of a trial. Another problem is evident if small numbers of products are tried. With the large number of garments now available it is important that each different type of garment is assessed as small numbers further limit the value of the results.

The trial I am going to describe (Fader *et al.*, 1986) was designed to overcome these problems. A very wide range of garments was chosen to be tried by patients coming from a variety of settings. Patients would assess the performance of garments that were suited to them and in this way it was hoped that it would be possible to classify patients requiring incontinence garments. This, in turn, would assist health-care workers in the appropriate prescription of these products.

There is little information available about the relationship between the constituents and design of incontinence garments and how they perform clinically. Malone-Lee (1984) described the technology of incontinence garments and the factors involved in their manufacture which may influence their performance. In order to examine this relationship the trial was carried out in conjunction with a technical study. In this way it was possible to determine what aspects of the garment, including their design and constituents were most likely to determine their clinical performance (Fader *et al.*, 1986).

Methods

Sample

Patients known to the Incontinence Clinic at St Pancras Hospital and using incontinence garments were asked to co-operate with the study. In order to ensure that the patient population came from a variety of settings the total population was to be divided equally between subjects living in their own homes, subjects on long-stay geriatric hospital wards and subjects resident in Part III homes. Informed consent was obtained from the patient, or from the carer if the patient's cognitive function was impaired.

Volumes Study

In order to estimate the severity of incontinence suffered by each subject a volumes study was done. Each subject or carer was supplied with enough pre-weighed pads (Cumfie Range by Vernon Carus) to last three days and asked to collect these in individual polyethylene bags after use. They also kept a record of when the pads were changed. At the end of the three days the pads were collected and weighed to estimate the volumes lost.

Group Selection

On completion of this initial assessment a decision was made as to which group the subject should be entered into. This was based on the information available from the subject questionnaire and the volumes study and as a result of the expressed preference of the subject or carer following inspection of representative products from each of the groups (see below).

Subjects recruited

137 subjects were recruited into the study.
    Group 1   33 females and one male entered Group 1. Their median

age was 74 with a range of 25 to 91. All except for one lady living in a Part III home were living in their own homes in the community.

Group 2   101 subjects entered into Group 2. There were 79 females and 22 males. Their median age was 81.5 years with a range of 58 to 105. Three of the men lived in the community, the remainder of this group lived in one of six long-stay hospital wards or five Part III homes being cared for by nurses or care assistants.

Group 3   47 subjects were entered into Group 3, 45 of whom were also in Group 2. There were 39 females and 8 males with a median age of 81 and a range of 68 to 105.

Procedure

On entry to the study information was obtained about the subject's medical state, the nature and size of their incontinence problem and their general social circumstances. All subjects underwent two tests of cognitive function, the Royal College of Physicians Mental Test Score (RCP) and the Complex Practical Skills Task of the Silver Mental Test Score (CPST). The RCP score is marked out of 34 with normal elderly people scoring from 28 to 34. A score of 18 or below is usually incompatible with independent existence (Hodkinson, 1973). The CPST score tests perception, visuo-spatial orientation and manipulative ability and is marked out of 16. A score of 10 or below would indicate a very significant disability (Silver, 1972), The Norton score was also recorded. This nursing assessment is marked out of 20 and scores below 14 are associated with an increased risk of pressure sore development (Norton et al., 1975).

Garment Selection

In 1982 all the companies marketing incontinence garments in the UK were contacted and asked to describe their products. Twenty-six different products were selected for the study, with the aim of covering as wide a range of garments as possible. Some duplication of garment types was necessary because of widely varying materials and the possibility that this might affect performance. The products selected are listed in Appendix A using a classification based on their design. All garments have a non-woven coverstock and a polyethylene backing unless stated to the contrary. Figures 1–7 illustrate the basic types of garments selected for the trial.

Garment Classification

The garments were classified into three groups, using the advice of the manufacturers:

Group 1   Garments for light incontinence.
Group 2   Garments for heavy daytime incontinence.
Group 3   Garments for heavy night-time incontinence.

It was thought that a fourth group might be necessary to cater for those subjects with moderate incontinence. This would have contained garments from both Group 1 and Group 2. However in practice, all subjects in this group rejected the larger pads, and were willing to try only those in Group 1.

Questionnaire

Subjects were asked to try each garment in their group for approximately seven days and the garments were offered in random order. The subject's or carer's assessment of the garment was obtained by questionnaire. Refusal to try a product or premature withdrawal was noted and at the end of the trial the subjects stated which garment they preferred.

When subjects were resident in a Part III home or a hospital ward the information usually had to be obtained from nurses or care assistants. In these circumstances a group response was obtained from a minimum quorum of three staff. Individual subject responses were impractical because of the mental state of such patients.

Results

Statistical Analysis

All parametric data was analysed by comparison of the difference between means using Student's t-test. Non-parametric data was analysed using contingency tables and chi-squared test. Where appropriate the Fisher exact probability test was used in place of the chi-squared test.

Subject Analysis

The data obtained from individual group members has been analysed and detailed in Tables 1 and 2. Very significant differences can be

Table 1   Characteristics of patients in Groups 1 and 2

	Group 1 Mean (SD)	Group 2 Mean (SD)	p value
Age (years)	70 (17)	82 (8)	0.0005
Norton score	16 (1)	13 (2)	0.0005
RCP score	30 (3)	7.5 (9.5)	0.0005
CPST score	15 (2)	3 (5)	0.0005

Table 2   Characteristics of patients in Groups 2 and 3

	Group 2 Mean (SD)	Group 3 Mean (SD)	p value
Age (years)	82 (8)	83 (8)	NS
Norton score	13 (2)	13 (2)	NS
RCP score	7.5 (9.5)	6 (9)	NS
CPST score	3 (5)	2.5 (4)	NS

SD = Standard deviation.
NS = No significant difference.
Maximum Norton score = 20.
Maximum RCP score = 34.
Maximum CPST score = 16.

shown between Groups 1 and 2. Differences between Groups 2 and 3 are less marked but this is to be expected.

The subjects in Group 1 tended to live in the community in their own homes, they were self-caring and ambulant. Those in Groups 2 and 3 lived in hospital wards and Part III homes being cared for by nurses or care assistants. They were a very dependent population that was older with significantly higher volume losses ($p < 0.0005$), (Figure 8). Groups 2 and 3 demonstrated significantly poorer scores on mental testing, tests of practical skills, mobility and independence ($p < 0.0005$).

Subjects in Groups 2 and 3 were significantly less mobile than those in Group 1 ($p < 0.0005$). There was a correlation between mobility and the Group selected ($p < 0.0005$).

There was no significant difference between the three groups in the frequency of episodes of incontinence during the day (mean = 2–3 episodes/day), but Group 2 had more episodes of nocturnal incontinence than those in Group 1 ($p < 0.0005$). Patients in Group 1 assessed themselves as less wet when incontinent than did those in Groups 2 and 3 ($p < 0.05$). 'Stress' and 'Urge' (as opposed to 'Passive' and 'Immobility') were symptoms more commonly associated with incontinence in Group 1 than in Groups 2 and 3 ($p < 0.0005$).

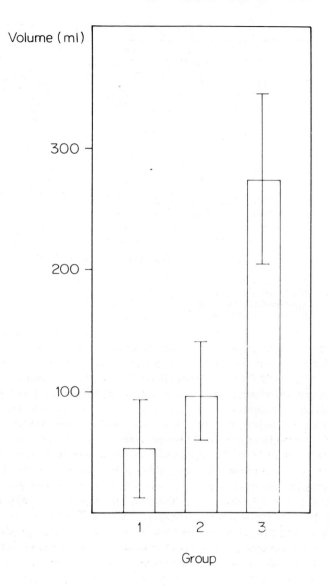

Figure 8   Mean urine loss (see volumes study). Error
bars = 1 standard deviation

The number of patients reporting faecal incontinence was less in Group 1 than in other groups ($p < 0.0005$).

Patients in Group 1 visited the lavatory more often, were quicker in getting there and could 'hang on' to their urine for longer periods than those in the other Groups ($p < 0.0005$). Similarly Group 1 patients required much less assistance in visiting the lavatory ($p < 0.005$). Patients in Group 1 were less likely to wear an incontinence garment all of the time and more likely to use it only on going out or during other specific activities ($p < 0.0005$). They were also more likely to change a pad because it was damp as opposed to wet ($p < 0005$). Patients in Groups 2 and 3 were more likely to change or have the pad changed because it was wet ($p < 0.0005$).

In all groups there was a predominance of women. This may reflect the higher proportion of women in the aged population, the higher incidence of incontinence in the female population, and the smaller numbers of men who are considered best suited to incontinence pads.

Garment Performance

Pads

The patients' and carers' responses to the question 'How did you like this pad' were recorded on an ordinal scale.

The Kanga Single pad received the most favourable response in Group 1, whether it was used with the Kanga Lady pants or the Sandralux pants. The Molinea Plus D (small) received a much less favourable response ($p < 0.05$) (Figure 9).

In Group 2 the Tenaform Normal was very favourably received with the Slipad and Cumfie large being well received in some Part III homes. The Kanga Standard, Molinea Plus D, Urocare, Incocare, Cumfie (medium) and Incontinette were considered less than 'alright' by over 50 per cent of respondents ($p < 0.0005$) (Figure 10).

In Group 3 the Tenaform Super was the most popular product with the Tenders being well received in one ward and two Part III homes ($p < 0.01$) (Figure 11).

Pants

The responses to the pants were measured on a similar ordinal scale to that described above. In Group 1 the Sandralux pants were the most

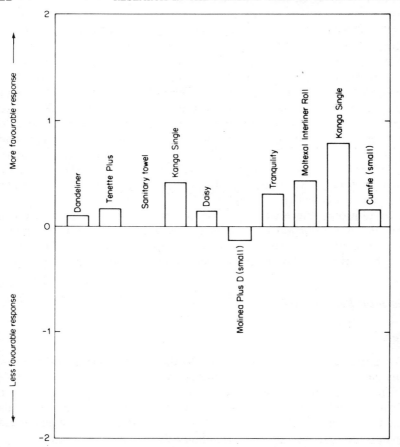

Figure 9   An analysis of the answers of Group 1 respondents to the question, 'How do you feel about the pad generally?'

popular and the Moltexal pants the least popular but the variations in responses in this group were not statistically significant (Figure 12).

In Group 2 the differences in response were highly significant ($p < 0.0005$). The pants supplied with the Tenaform Normal, IPS Interliner, and the Molinea Plus D were well received whereas the Doublet pants and the Urocare pants were not liked. The Doublet pants were found to fit less well ($p < 0.0005$) and were less comfortable ($p < 0.0005$) than other pants used in Group 2. The Urocare pants were also considered to be less comfortable than others in the Group (Figure 13).

The Sandralux pants, Tranquility pants, and Kanga Lady pants were considered significantly more attractive than others tried by the respondents in Group 1 ($p < 0.01$). The Doublet pants were considered

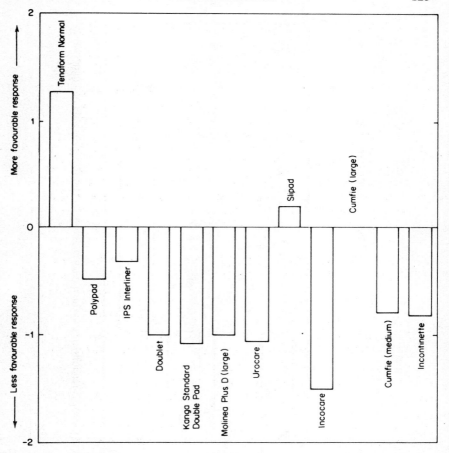

Figure 10 An analysis of the answers of Group 2 respondents to the question, 'How do you feel about the pad generally?'

unattractive by a significant number of Group 2 respondents ($p < 0.0005$).

Structure

The views of the patients or carers on the structure of the pads were assessed using the question: 'Was the structure of the pad satisfactory/ not satisfactory?' The response to this question was qualified with a description of what was considered wrong with the pad.

The Kanga single pad produced a favourable response even though

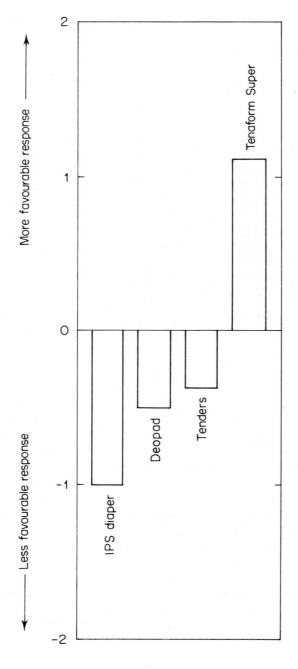

Figure 11   An analysis of the answers of Group 3 respondents to the question, 'How do you feel about the pad generally?'

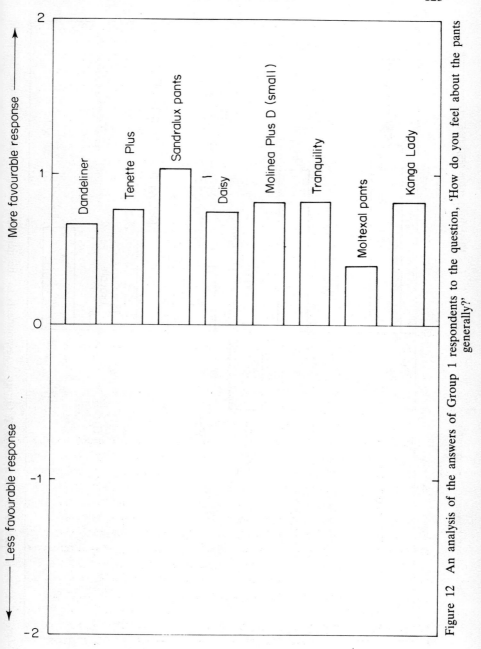

Figure 12 An analysis of the answers of Group 1 respondents to the question, 'How do you feel about the pants generally?'

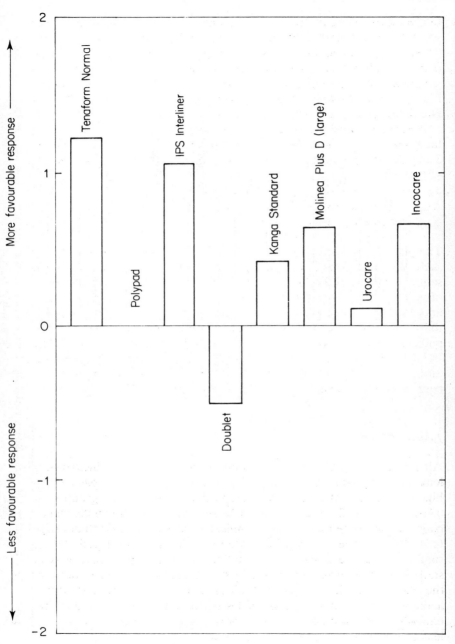

Figure 13 An analysis of the answers of Group 2 respondents to the question, 'How do you feel about the pants

tested twice. (With the Kanga Lady pants and with Henley's Sandralux pants.) It was found to be the most satisfactory pad in Group 1 ($p < 0.001$). The Tranquility pad and Brevet Moltexal Interliner Role appeared to get closest to the ideal size. The sanitary towel was frequently judged to be too short and too narrow, whereas the Tenette Plus pad and Molinea Plus D pad were considered too wide. The Dandeliner pad was often judged to be too thick.

In Group 2 the Tenaform Normal pad was considered satisfactory far more often than any of the other products ($p < 0.001$). In Group 3 the Tenaform Super pad attracted similarly favourable responses ($p < 0.005$).

Absorbency

The patients, or their carers, were asked to rate the absorbency of the pads as, 'Too great', 'About right' or 'Too little'. In Group 1 the sanitary towel and the Molinea Plus D pad were rated 'Too little' more often than others ($p < 0.0005$). In Group 2 the absorbency of the Slipad and Tenaform Normal pad were frequently rated 'About right' whereas that of the Incocare, Polypad, Doublet, Molinea Plus D, and Urocare pads were rated as 'Too little' more frequently than others ($p < 0.0005$). In Group 3 50 per cent rated the Tenders, and 75 per cent the Tenaform Super, as 'About right'; 25 per cent rated the Tenaform Super as containing more absorbent than was necessary.

Leakage

All of the pads in Group 1 were found to have a very low incidence of leakage. The sanitary towel, Daisy and Cumfie (small) pads had a higher incidence of occasional leakage than others in the group ($p < 0.05$). In Group 2 The Tenaform Normal, Slipad and Cumfie (large) pads were reported as leaking significantly less frequently than others ($p < 0.005$). The Incocare and Molinea Plus D (large) pads leaked significantly more frequently ($p < 0.005$). In Group 3 there was no statistically significant difference in the incidence of leakage between the pads though it occurred with all of them. The commonest sites of leakage in all groups were the sides of the pads but in Group 2 the back and the front of the pads were frequently recorded as sites of leakage.

Confidence

Group 1 patients felt substantially more confident with the Kanga Lady garment but less confident when wearing the sanitary towel or Daisy garment ($p < 0.0005$). In Groups 2 and 3 the differences in confidence induced by different garments were not significant.

Comfort

For all groups, the differences in assessment of the comfort of individual products were not statistically significant. All products were considered to be uncomfortable when wet. When dry they were usually assessed as comfortable or tolerable.

Ease of application

The question 'Did you have any difficulties putting on the garment or taking it off?' could be answered, 'Yes' or 'No'. This produced significant differences in responses in Group 2 only. The Doublet, Slipad and Incontinette garments proved difficult to put on and take off more often than others in the group ($p < 0.0005$).

The question 'Did you have any difficulties putting the pad in position?' was also answered, 'Yes' or 'No'. In Group 1 the Dandeliner garment caused difficulties most often ($p < 0.005$). In Group 2 The Incontinette, Slipad, Urocare, Kanga Standard and Kanga Doublet caused difficulties more often than other garments ($p < 0.005$). Group 3 responses were not significantly different.

When asked about the ease of removing the wet pad the only significant response differences were found in Group 2 where the Kanga Standard and Urocare pads were rated distinctly more difficult to remove when wet ($p < 0.005$). Many carers commented on the unpleasantness of putting their hands into a patient's wet pouch.

Holding pad in position

In Group 1 the Kanga Lady pants were substantially more efficient at holding the pad in position than other pants were ($p < 0.05$). The Sandralux pants were less efficient than the Kanga Lady pants in holding the same pad in position. In Group 2 the pants used with the Tenaform Normal, Kanga Standard and Urocare garments maintained the position of the pad more efficiently than others ($p < 0.001$). Group 3 garments showed no significant differences in their abilities to maintain the pads in position.

No significant differences or variations were found in odour or skin health. None of the products appeared to alter the patient's life-style or choice of clothing. No problems were encountered with washing any of the pants.

Discussion

It would seem from the results of this study that patients requiring incontinence garments should be divided into three groups. The factors determining the grouping are the mobility and independence of the patient. The symptomatology, apart from describing nocturnal incontinence seems to be less important in group selection.

Patients who are mobile and independent require garments suitable for light incontinence. Their needs are well met from the range of garments tried in Group 1. These patients tended to prefer small pads even if they were considered quite heavily incontinent and would seem to prefer to change their pads more often rather than wear a large, bulky pad. Discretion was considered to be very important by subjects in Group 1 and many of the comments that were recorded on the questionnaire referred to the excessive bulkiness of some of the pads, for example:

'Felt like riding a horse'
'Like a sack of coal'
'Made me walk with my legs further apart'

The needs of patients in Group 1 seemed to be well met from the range of pads that they tried. The most successful pad being the Kanga single pad which, it is interesting to note, was also the cheapest pad in the range. The Sandralux pants or the Kanga Lady pants were used with this pad and both were very favourably received.

None of the plastic backed pads in Group 1 did very well. It would seem that there is room for improvement with these pads. The sanitary towel was not successful and should not be considered as an alternative to a purpose-made incontinence pad. The pads which incorporated hydrogels were not well received and some subjects complained about the pads feeling slimey or porridge-like when wet. These pads were also considerably more expensive than other pads in this range.

Patients who are immobile and/or dependent on others for care require incontinence garments suitable for heavy daytime incontinence

(Group 2) and for heavy night-time incontinence (Group 3) if this is also a problem.

Despite the fact that the volumes lost by patients in Group 2 were surprisingly low (mean 96 ml (SD 60)) very few garments could cope successfully without leaking, although some manufacturers claimed that their pads could hold several times this amount. The needs of the patients in Group 2 were generally very poorly met by the range of garments tried.

One pad did outstandingly well — the Tenaform Normal. The Slipad also proved popular and effective, but some nursing staff disliked the fact that they were so similar to babies nappies. They also proved difficult to change and it was thought that this could discourage staff from toileting patients. As the Slipad was effective in preventing leakage some staff thought that patients could be left in wet pads for excessive lengths of time.

Garments using the marsupial principle did badly in Group 2. The pads were frequently considered to be too small and staff commented about the unpleasantness of removing soaked pads from the pouches. It was also commented that if some subjects were faecally incontinent the pants were then heavily soiled and difficult and nasty to clean. It is interesting to note that the marsupial principle did very well in Group 1 and it would seem reasonable that removing your own wet pad from your pouch is very different to removing someone else's.

The wing folded diapers did not attract favourable responses in any of the homes or wards. Problems with applying the pad correctly were noted in particular.

Most pants in Group 2 were well liked. However, front-opening pants were found to be much more difficult to put on than pull-on pants, despite the fact that these were supposed to be easier to apply for dependent subjects.

Immobile and/or dependent patients with heavy night-time incontinence are best managed using garments in Group 3. In general there was a variable response to night pads in hospital wards, though in Part III homes they were readily accepted. Nursing staff on some wards found night pads in general more difficult to change than bedpads and also commented on difficulties observing patients' pressure areas. The most successful garment from the range tried in Group 3 was the Tenaform Super. It would seem that garments for night-time incontinence may not be ideal for all patients and that alternatives, such as reusable bedpads may be better for some patients.

Problems Conducting Clinical Trials of Products

Nurses are under increasing pressure to assess the products that they are using, for clinical and cost effective reasons. However, clinical trials are not to be undertaken lightly. The length of time necessary is frequently underestimated; this trial took two years to complete by one research nurse full time (one year was estimated). If the nurse is involved in research part-time the needs of her patients will always take priority over the trial and consequently the time taken will be even longer.

It is seductive to be asked to try a few products by a representative from a company, but it must be remembered that uncontrolled, *ad hoc* trials rarely yield any useful results. Novelty is a very powerful factor and patients trying a couple of new products and receiving extra attention are likely to want to 'please' the researcher. Even very small 'just a couple of boxes' trials take some time and unless you know the results will be worth the effort they are usually not worth doing.

Companies themselves are becoming more involved in conducting their own trials with their own products. These promotional trials should not be confused with research. It is obvious that with a considerable amount of company input results will be biased. Do not expect that a company will go through all the expense and effort for nothing; the results are extremely likely to be in the companies' favour.

Clinical trials performed by independent bodies are essential to provide the patient with the most effective product. Any new drug is assessed for safety and for efficacy. It is high time that the same thing happened to aids used by patients. The cost to industry will be high, as clinical trials will have to be funded, but unless a new product is put on trial it is impossible to assess whether money is being wasted, false economies made or whether the patient will benefit or suffer. This trial demonstrated that the most expensive product is not necessarily the best; and sometimes the cheapest is. However, similar products can perform very differently and without clinical trials there is no way of knowing whether a cheap reproduction will be as effective as the original.

Conclusions

The type of incontinence garment a patient will require seems to be dependent on the patient's mobility and independence rather than the symptoms or degree of incontinence.

In our study the Kanga single pad and Sandralux or Kanga Lady pants are recommended for mobile, independent patients. These patients require small discreet pads rather than large bulky ones. The Tenaform Normal and Stretch pants were found to be by far the most satisfactory garment for immobile and/or dependent patients. For patients with heavy night-time incontinence the Tenaform Super and Stretch pants are recommended. These would provide a minimum range of incontinence garments, but none were acceptable to all patients in their groups. A wider range is preferable to suit individual needs.

References

Bainton, D., Blanin, J. B. and Shepherd, A. M. (1982). Pads and pants for urinary incontinence. *Br. Med. J.*, **285**, 419–420.

Fader, M. J., Barnes K. E., Malone-Lee, J. and Cottenden, A. (1986). Incontinence Garments — Results of a DHSS Study. *Health Equipment Information No. 159*. DHSS, London.

Health Services Supplies Council (1984). A market appraisal of the supply of incontinence pads to the National Health Service, 1–10.

Hodkinson, H. M. (1973). Mental impairment in the elderly. *J. Roy. Coll. Phys.*, **17**, 4, 305–317.

Malone-Lee, J. (1984). The technology of absorbents. *Care*, **4**, 2, 22–28.

Malone-Lee, J., McCreery, M. and Exton-Smith, A. N. (1982). A community study of the performance of incontinence garments. *DHSS Aids Assessment Programme*.

Masterton, G., Holloway, E. M. and Timbury, G. C. (1980). The prevalence of incontinence in local authority homes for the elderly. *Health Bulletin*, **38**, 2, 62–64.

Milne, J. S. (1976). Prevalence of incontinence in the elderly age groups, in F. L. Willington (Ed.), *Incontinence in the Elderly*, pp. 9–21. Academic Press, London.

Norton, C. (1982). The effects of urinary incontinence in women. *Int. Rehab. Med.*, **4**, 9–14.

Norton, D., McLaren, R. and Exton-Smith, A. N. (1975). *An Investigation of Geriatric Nursing Problems in Hospital*. Churchill Livingstone, Edinburgh.

Schofield, D. and Schofield, D. (1981). Stress incontinence — the solution solidified. *Nursing Times*, 28 October, 1885–1886.

Sheperd, A. M. and Blanin, J. (1980). A clinical trial of pants and pads used for urinary incontinence. *Nursing Times*, 5 June, 1015–1016.

Silver, C. P. S. (1972). Simple methods of testing ability in geriatric patients. *Geront. Clin.*, **14**, 110–112.

Tam, G., Knox, J. G. and Adamson, M. (1978). A cost effectiveness trial of incontinence pads. *Nursing Times*, 20 July 1198–1200.

Thomas, T. M., Plymat, K. R., Blanin, J. and Meade T. (1980). Prevalence of urinary incontinence. *Br. Med. J.*, **281**, 1243–1245.

Watson, A. C. (1980). A trial of Molnlycke pants and diapers. *Nursing Times*, 5 June, 1017–1019.

Willington, F. L. (1969). Problems in urinary incontinence in the aged. *Geront. Clin.*, **11**, 330–356.
Willington, F. L., Lade, C. M. and Thomas, A. M. (1972). Marsupial pants for urinary incontinence. *Nursing Mirror*, **135**, 40–41.

Appendix A

Garment description	Garment name	Manufacturer
Pulp-filled pads	Dandeliner	Smith & Nephew
(Figure 1)	Tenette Plus	Molnlycke
Stretch pants	Tenaform Normal	Molnlycke
(Figure 2)	Tenaform Super	Molnlycke
	Molinea Plus-D (small)	Paul Hartmann
	Molinea Plus-D (large)	Paul Hartmann
	Cumfie (small)	Vernon Carus
	Cumfie (medium)	Vernon Carus
	Cumfie (large)	Vernon Carus
	IPS Interliner	IPS
	Polypad	Undercover
	Incocare Insert	Robinsons
Pulp-filled pads*	Standard (double)	Nicholas (Kanga)
(Figures 3 + 4)	Lady (single)	Nicholas (Kanga)
Pants + waterproof	Urocare (double)	IDC
pouch/pocket	Sandralux (single)	Henley's
(Figure 5)		
Wing-folded pads	Folded diaper	IPS
(Figure 7)	Deopad	LIC
Stretch pants	Doublet†	Nicholas (Kanga)
(Figure 2)		
Pads + super-absorbency	Tranquility*	Henley's
gels		
Special pants	Daisy	LIC
Adult all-in-one diapers	Tenders	Ancilla
(Figure 6)	Slipad	Peadouce
Sanitary pad	Stayfree (Super)	Johnson & Johnson
Subject's own pants		
Wing-folded pads	Incontinette	Ancilla
Adhesive tabs		
Wadding roll*	Moltexal Interliner	Brevet
Specially designed pants		

* No polyethylene backing
† Special front-opening pants

Research in the Nursing Care of Elderly People
Edited by P. Fielding
© 1987 John Wiley & Sons Ltd

CHAPTER 6

Prediction of Rehabilitation Success

PAULINE FIELDING

Introduction

Background to the Project

This study was carried out in response to a need to use scarce resources in the most effective way. The scarce resource in question was a ten bedded rehabilitation ward which was part of an acute geriatric department in a large London teaching hospital. The department exercised an age-related admissions policy which determined that any patient over the age of 75 years who was not already being treated by a hospital consultant, was admitted under the care of a geriatrician. Such patients were admitted into a general pool of beds on medical and, sometimes, surgical wards. They could broadly be classified into three groups — those suffering from an acute illness who would recover uneventfully and return to their homes; those who were so disabled as to become unable to function outside an institution and so became 'long stay' and were transferred elsewhere; and those who, after recovering from the acute phase of their illness, seemed inappropriately placed on an acute ward and needed more intensive rehabilitation before they could return to their home in the community.

It was important to be able to identify this latter group of patients in order to transfer them to the rehabilitation ward as it afforded a more suitable environment in several respects than the general wards. The nurse : patient ratio, at 1 : 0.8 was considerably higher than in the other wards. The toilet : patient ratio was 1 : 5 compared with 1 : 10 on the general wards and no bed was more than 40 feet from a toilet whereas in the general wards only a small proportion of beds were within such a distance. These two factors which are of crucial significance in rehabilitation, combined with a more homely, domestic environment, ensured the use of this ward to its best advantage in the care of elderly patients needing substantial input from nurses, physiotherapists and occupational therapists.

It is generally recognized that rehabilitation is labour intensive and time consuming and some have also recognized that it is not always undertaken rationally. Brocklehurst *et al.* (1978), writing about stroke patients, point out that a patient is more likely to receive physiotherapy if the stroke is severe, regardless of the premorbid state of health, age, sex or level of mobility. Indeed, Brocklehurst and his colleagues suggest that stroke patients continue to use resources long after they have passed the optimal point of recovery. In times of financial stringency, this is a situation that the health service can ill afford and more recently Prescott *et al.* (1982) have suggested that clinicians might consider applying available resources to those patients who are most likely to derive maximum benefit from them. The problem then becomes one of prediction — who will benefit most from the scarce resources available?

Literature Review

Development of Predictive Measures

In everyday clinical practice, predictions of recovery are made all the time but such judgements, whether successful or unsuccessful, rest more on intuition and experience than on any objective or systematic assessment. However, some attempts at systematic objectivity have been made and are worth noting.

In 1960, Bruell and Simon suggested the possibility of developing objective methods of prediction. They questioned whether or not there was a basis in fact to the belief that hemiplegic patients who received physiotherapy early after the event would recover more successfully than those who received it somewhat later. They studied two samples of 40 hemiplegic patients — two failure groups consisting of patients who, in spite of treatment, remained wheelchair bound and two recovery groups who progressed from being wheelchair bound to being fully independent on discharge home. From examination of hospital records they were able to report that in both samples, the patients who recovered received physiotherapy significantly earlier in the illness phase, than did the patients who failed to recover.

However, while the time of onset of physiotherapy could explain their results, Bruell and Simon point out that the failure group may have been more disabled than the recovery group and independent measures of disability were needed. Using the same samples of patients, age and systolic blood pressure on admission were noted and subsequently found to differentiate between the groups in that the failure group were older and had higher systolic blood pressures than the recovery group. Clearly then, the performance of the failure group could be attributable to greater disablement (as measured by age and systolic blood pressure) rather than to delayed physiotherapy.

Leaving aside the question as to whether age and systolic blood pressure are valid indicators of disability, Bruell and Simon went on to combine these and time of instigation of physiotherapy to produce a composite score which successfully differentiated the failure and recovery groups. The authors themselves discuss several shortcomings of the work but despite its limitations it remains a significant study in the development of objective predictors.

Peszczynski (1961) was also concerned with the need to predict recovery in elderly hemiplegic patients and although he accepted that the patient's goal was functional recovery, he focused on those clinical prognostic factors which he argued were essential in any prediction of level of independence. These clinical factors are itemized in Table 1. Unfortunately he presents no empirical data to support these factors which, he admits, are based on his own clinical impressions and personal experience. However, in recent research, clinical factors have been related to functional outcome in attempts to develop predictive tools.

The Bristol Prognostic Score was developed by Wade et al. (1983)

Table 1   Clinical prognostic factors in cerebrovascular accidents. (Peszczynski, 1961)

Prolonged bowel incontinence
Urinary incontinence
Flexion contracture of the hemiplegic knee
Type of motor involvement
Sensory involvement in hemiplegia
Hemianopia
Pain in hemiplegia
Aphasia
Mental derangements
Motivation
Body image

using five clinical variables in their assessment of 83 stroke patients (see
Table 2), using the Barthel Index as a measure of outcome. Of those
patients who survived to six months, they were able to predict recovery
to within five points in 55 per cent of patients and to within 10 points
in 72 per cent of patients.

Table 2   The Bristol Prognostic Score clinical
variables

Urinary incontinence
Motor deficit in arm
Sitting balance
Hemianopia
Age

The Guy's Hospital Prognostic Score (Allen, 1984a) achieved similar
results in a sample of 137 patients (see Table 3). Allen (1984b)
concludes that with regard to cerebrovascular accidents (CVAs), the
relevant prognostic factors are those pertaining to the site and size of
brain lesion together with the patient's underlying pathology.

Table 3   The Guy's Hospital prognostic score

Complete paralysis of worst limb
Higher cerebral dysfunction and hemianopia and hemiplegia
Drowsy or comatose after 24 hours
Age
Loss of consciousness at onset of stroke
Uncomplicated hemiparesis (no higher cerebral dysfunction or hemianopia)

Development of Functional Assessment

Since the beginnings of geriatric medicine in the 1940s there has been
a growing recognition of the importance of functional assessment, i.e.
what the person can or cannot do for himself, over and against any
clinical prognosis. Hall (1976) points out that because multiple pathology is so common in the elderly, it would not be unusual for an
elderly person to have 20–30 problems, but for only a proportion of
these would he or she desire treatment. Consequently, suggests Hall,
the assessment of disability should be focused in 'behavioural terms'
rather than in terms of pathology or diagnosis even though these latter
may have an important role in correcting the diminished behavioural

performance. In other words, functional assessment is of primary importance.

There are now a variety of tools with which to assess functional ability and which focus on particular functions or client groups. One of the earliest and perhaps best known is the Barthel Index (Mahoney and Barthel, 1965). It is a 10-item index (see Table 4) designed for use on patients with a neuromuscular or musculo-skeletal disorder. The values assigned to each item are based on the time and amount of physical assistance required if a patient is unable to perform the activity and some activities are weighted more heavily than others depending on their significance for independent living. Since this early work by Mahoney and Barthel, many studies have been published which have used quantitative assessments of performance on various activities of daily living (ADLs) (Adler, Brown and Acton, 1980; Carroll, 1968; Dinnerstein, Lowenthal and Dexter, 1965; Granger, Albrecht and Hamilton, 1979; Katz *et al.*, 1970; Lawton and Brody, 1969; Pfeiffer, 1976; Sheikh *et al.*, 1979).

Table   4   The   Barthel   Index.
(Mahoney and Barthel, 1965)

1	Feeding	6	Walking
2	Transfers	7	Stairs
3	Personal Toilet	8	Dressing
4	On/off toilet	9	Bowels
5	Bathing	10	Bladder
	Score from 0–100		

The advantages of functional assessment are at least threefold. Firstly, the use of a functional assessment tool does not depend on a high level of medical knowledge — what is required is an ability to observe and rate performance. It is thus a valuable multidisciplinary tool which can provide a common language not only between those caring for the patient but between the patient and his carers. Secondly, functional assessment can provide a means of measuring progress and of evaluating particular types of treatment. Such recording of progress also provides valuable feedback to the patient which helps to focus effort and stimulate motivation. Thirdly, functional assessment can help to identify deficiencies in performance which will impede the attainment of independence. In all, an accurate and objective functional assessment can lift the patient's treatment programme out of the realms of subjectivity and provide a focus for the patient's and team's efforts.

However, as with any measuring instrument, validity and reliability must be considered. The notion of validity with regard to functional assessment relates to how well any tests carried out in assessment, correlate to what the patient has to do in normal circumstances at home. Indeed, it may not be possible to select activities which are familiar and relevant to all patients who return to a variety of home circumstances. The plethora of rating instruments which have been developed may be one indication of this problem. Another important consideration is whether a single activity such as dressing or making transfers can be isolated from other activities in any meaningful way. It could be argued that the ability to move from wheelchair to toilet is of little significance if the patient is unable to dress himself. Reliability is also a crucial issue — do two observers testing the same patient arrive at the same test score? Carroll (1968) reports an inter-rater reliability of 90 per cent in his study but points out that this does not mean that others using the method in other institutions will obtain the same results.

Role of Mental Status

It has long been recognized that there is evidence for a correlation between physical and mental status (Kahn and Goldberg, 1960), and Denham and Jeffreys (1972) and Qureshi and Hodkinson (1974) both demonstrated the usefulness of a mental status questionnaire in planning a realistic rehabilitation programme. Mental clarity is obviously an advantage in any treatment programme but is perhaps particularly important in situations where a carry-over of learning is required. For example, in Stewart (1980) an improvement in dressing ability was highly significantly correlated with higher mental test scores. Stewart argues that dressing is an activity learned at an early age and is not a natural instinct like walking. When this ability is lost, it is the patient with the higher mental test score who is able to relearn it.

Testing mental status presents problems, however, particularly in a frail, elderly population. Peszczynski (1961) points out that some of the confusion demonstrated by recently admitted hemiplegic patients may be the transient consequences of brain oedema, or may reflect a difficulty in adjustment to new surroundings. Kahn and Goldberg's mental status questionnaire (MSQ) (1960) is fairly simple and not too taxing for elderly patients. Denham and Jeffreys (1972) and Roth and Hopkins (1953) developed longer questionnaires but as Stewart (1980) argued, prolonged questioning can lead to a loss of concentration and enthusiasm and may produce misleading results.

Few of the studies mentioned thus far deal with a general elderly population. Much of the literature relates to either hemiplegic patients or amputees. A notable exception is Stewart (1980) and his study will now be reviewed in more detail.

Using an ADL score modified from Carroll (1968), Stewart rated 61 admissions to a geriatric rehabilitation unit on admission and subsequently every four weeks until a final decision was made to classify the patients into three discharge groups — Continuing Care, Residential Home for the Elderly, or their own home. In addition to the modified ADL score, Kahn and Goldberg's MSQ (1960) was included.

The construction of the ADL score and the MSQ are shown in the appendix. The weighting of ADL items indicates the relative importance of various factors in relation to the final discharge of the patient from the rehabilitation unit. Thus Stewart observed that the control of bowels, bladder and the ability to walk were, excluding MSQ, the most important factors in determining discharge.

Stewart's results show that, of the 61 patients (26 men, 35 women), 20 per cent went home; 28 per cent were discharged to a Residential Home; 52 per cent were transferred to Continuing Care. Patients with low scores (less than 50) made little progress and tended to be placed in Continuing Care wards. Those with high scores (more than 80) were able to leave the hospital quickly. The greatest improvement occurred in a group with middle range scores (50–80) and Stewart suggests that these are the patients who have benefited most from the facilities of the rehabilitation unit. He argues from these data for selective admission of such patients in order to make the most of restricted facilities.

This study is an attempt to use Stewart's findings in a different setting in order to test the usefulness of the ADL score in identifying those patients who will benefit most from rehabilitation facilities.

Hypotheses

The following hypotheses were tested:
1 There will be no difference in the amount of progress made between patients who score within or outside Stewart's rehabilitation range of 50–80 points.
2 There will be no relationship between scoring within Stewart's rehabilitation range on admission and making progress.
3 Patients will not be differentiated on admission scores in terms of final placement.

4 Patients will not be differentiated on discharge scores in terms of final placement.
5 There will be no relationship between MSQ score on admission and making progress.
6 There will be no relationship between MSQ score on admission and final discharge group.

Method

Sample

The sample of patients was drawn from the population of male and female patients under the care of two geriatricians at a large London teaching hospital. The sample identified were those patients who, in the opinion of the multidisciplinary team, were in need of rehabilitation. For some patients, this was on admission to hospital, for others it was following recovery from an acute event such as a chest infection. Referrals for rehabilitation were made most often at the weekly multidisciplinary case conference.

Eighty-three patients were included in the study, of whom eight died and one was transferred to another hospital. The data relate, therefore, to 74 patients (12 men, 62 women) whose ages ranged from 69–101 years, with a mean age of 81.6 years.

Design

Initial assessment following referral for rehabilitation was repeated at fortnightly intervals until final placement.

Instruments

Stewart's ADL assessment scale (see Appendix).
Kahn and Goldberg's MSQ.

In addition to the above assessment tools, a patient profile was completed on the first assessment.

Procedure

Each patient was seen within 24 hours of referral and information was obtained by personal interview, formal assessment, from medical and nursing notes and by discussion with relevant staff members. Those patients who scored within Stewart's rehabilitation range of 50–80 points were transferred to the rehabilitation ward whenever possible. A note was made of the final discharge group of each patient, these being either their own home, Part III Social Services Residential Accommodation or Continuing Care in a long-stay ward.

Results

Inter-rater Reliability

Inter-rater reliability between the four researchers involved was established at 85 per cent.

Final Discharge Groups

Of the 74 patients finally studied, 54 per cent (40 patients) went home; 16 per cent (12 patients) were discharged to a Part III home and 30 per cent (22 patients) were transferred to Continuing Care.

Reason for Admission

Of the 74 patients studied, 58 per cent (43 patients) were admitted to hospital with an acute condition. Of these 60 per cent (26 patients) went home, 17 per cent (7 patients) were discharged to a Part III home and 23 per cent (10 patients) were transferred to Continuing Care (see Table 5). The remainder (31 patients) were admitted to hospital ostensibly for 'assessment and/or rehabilitation'. Of these, 45 per cent (14 patients) went home, 16 per cent (5 patients) were discharged to a Part III home and 39 per cent (12 patients) were transferred to Continuing Care. A chi-square Test of Association showed no significant relationship between reason for admission and final placement.

Table 5 Association between reason for admission and final discharge group

	Final discharge group		
Reason for admission	Home	Part III	Continuing Care
Acute event	26	7	10
Assessment/rehabilitation	14	5	12

Chi-squared = 2.27 (not significant).

Living Spouse

Only 11 per cent (8 patients) had a living spouse. Of these, seven patients went home and one was placed in Continuing Care.

Living Alone

A large proportion of patients, 66 per cent (49 patients) lived alone. Of these, 43 per cent (21 patients) went home, 24 per cent (12 patients) were discharged to a Part III home and 33 per cent (16 patients) were placed in Continuing Care.

Hypothesis 1 There will be no difference in the amount of progress made between patients who score within or outside Stewart's rehabilitation range of 50–80 points.

As can be seen from Table 6, there is no statistically significant difference in the amount of progress made between the two groups of patients. It is, however, clear that some patients outside the rehabilitation range are making substantial progress. A dot diagram (Figure 1) of progress plotted against admission scores shows that those patients who appear to make the most progress, score within a lower range of 25–55. This is statistically significant for patients whether in the rehabilitation ward or in the general wards (see Table 7).

Hypothesis 2 There will be no relationship between scoring within Stewart's rehabilitation range on admission and making progress.

Table 6   Amount of progress made within and outside Stewart's rehabilitation range

| Ward | Mean progress made | | T-value |
	Score 50–79	Score <50>80	
Rehabilitation	8.6 (*n*=19)	15.0 (*n*=23)	0.9 not sig.
General	6.8 (*n*=17)	14.5 (*n*=15)	1.2 not sig.

Table 7   Amount of progress made within and outside 25–55 ADL range

| Ward | Mean progress made | | T-value |
	Score 25–54	Score <25>55	
Rehabilitation	19.8 (*n*=19)	5.7 (*n*=23)	2.1 Sig. 5% level
General	21.4 (*n*=12)	3.8 (*n*=20)	2.8 Sig. 1% level

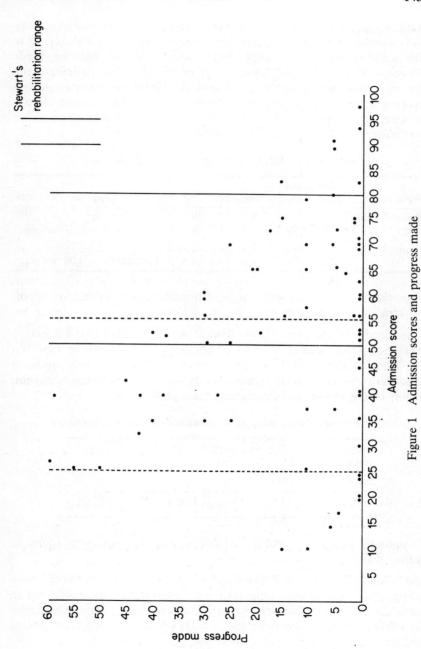

Figure 1 Admission scores and progress made

Table 8 shows that a Chi-square Test of Association revealed no statistically significant relationship between score on admission with regard to Stewart's rehabilitation range and whether or not patients made progress. Even using the lower range of 25–55 where patients made the most progress, there was no statistically significant association with making or not making progress. 'Progress' was defined as any change in score in an upwards direction. 'No progress' was defined as either no change in score or a reduction in score.

Table 8   ADL score on admission and progress

Ward	Admission score range	Progress	No progress
Rehabilitation	50–79	$n = 14$	$n = 5$
	<50>80	$n = 15$	$n = 8$ chi-squared = 0.07 not sig.
General	50–79	$n = 11$	$n = 6$
	<50>80	$n = 10$	$n = 5$ chi-squared = 0.06 not sig.

Hypothesis 3   Patients will not be differentiated on admission scores in terms of final placement.

Unrelated T Tests show (Table 9) that the Home and Part III groups were not differentiated in terms of admission ADL score as were not the Part III and Continuing Care groups. However, it was apparent that there was a statistically significant difference between the admission scores of the Home and Continuing Care groups.

Table 9   Mean admission scores and discharge groups

Home ($n=40$)	Part III ($n=12$)	Continuing Care ($n=22$)	T-value
56.98	51.17		0.9 Not sig.
	51.17	45.64	0.8 Not sig.
56.98		45.64	2.0 Sig. 5% level

Hypothesis 4   Patients will not be differentiated on discharge scores in terms of final placement.

On discharge, it was still not possible to differentiate between those going home and those going into residential care (see Table 10) in terms of their final discharge score. However, there was a statistically significant difference between the Part III and Continuing Care groups and between the Home and Continuing Care groups.

Table 10   Mean discharge scores and discharge groups

Home (n=40)	Part III (n=12)	Continuing Care (n=22)	T-value
74.5	67.8		0.9 Not sig.
	67.8	43.7	3.5 Sig. 2% level
74.5		43.7	5.5 Sig. 5% level

Hypothesis 5   There will be no relationship between MSQ score on admission and making or not making progress.

Table 11 shows that there is a statistically significant association between MSQ score on admission and the likelihood of making or not making progress. It seems that those patients who score 12 or more are more likely to make progress than not. However, there does not seem to be any such relationship between scoring 10 or less and the likelihood of not making progress.

Table 11   MSQ score on admission and progress

Admission MSQ score	Progress	No progress
$\geqslant 12$	33	9
$\leqslant 10$	17	15

Chi-squared = 4.3 Sig. 5% level.

Hypothesis 6   There will be no relationship between MSQ score on admission and final discharge groups.

It can be seen from Table 12 that there is a statistically significant association between MSQ score on admission and final discharge groups. Those patients scoring 12 or more are more likely to go home, whilst those scoring 10 or less are more likely to receive Continuing Care. However, on discharge, a chi-squared test of association showed that there was no relationship between MSQ score and final placement (chi-square = 4.6, 2 degrees of freedom).

Table 12   MSQ score on admission and final discharge group

Admission MSQ score	Home	Part III	Continuing Care
$\geqslant 12$	29	6	7
$\leqslant 10$	11	6	15

Chi-squared = 9.9 Sig. 1% level.

Predictors of Final Placement

A linear discriminant function analysis was carried out in order to see which items were the most powerful predictors of final placement. Four subsets of variables were used (see Table 13). Set I consisted of MSQ score and all individual ADL scores except the total score which is linearly dependent on the items included. Set II includes all Set I variables plus five additional variables. Set III and Set IV are the single variables of ADL total score and MSQ score respectively. The following data relate to 59 patients only as the remainder, selected at random, were used as a 'hold'out' sample for cross-validation purposes.

Table 13   Subsets of Variables used in linear discriminant analysis

Variable set	Names
I	Bowel function; bladder function; walking; dressing; toileting; feeding; wheelchair; stairs; mental status
II	Age; sex; living spouse; lives alone; stairs to climb; plus all variables in Set I
III	Total ADL score
IV	Mental status score

In the first two assessments, MSQ score was the most powerful discriminator. However, the situation altered as time went on (see Table 14). For Variable Set I, bladder function seemed to be one of the most useful predictors over all assessments whereas age was one of the most significant predictors for all assessments if Variable Set II was applied (see Table 15). Although this method seems promising, care must be exercised in its interpretation as there is a selective reduction in numbers with each assessment. Overall, the results obtained from the discriminant analysis are not satisfactory. There is no obvious discriminator which acts powerfully in every assessment (see Tables 16, 17) although Variable Set II seems to be the most likely candidate in comparison with the other three sets.

Discussion

Unfortunately, it has not been possible to replicate Stewart's findings and some explanation must be sought. The most obvious source of difference probably lies in the two samples. The patients in Stewart's

Table 14   Linear discriminant analysis: Variable Set I

Assessment no.	Percentage correct classification				No. patients
	Home	Part III	Continuing Care	Total	
1	58.3	50.0	61.5	57.6	59
2	58.3	60.0	38.5	54.2	59
3	81.0	80.0	60.0	75.0	36
4	55.6	50.0	83.3	63.2	19
5	85.7	66.7	100.0	83.3	12
6	75.0	100.0	100.0	87.5	8
7	100.0	50.0	100.0	75.0	4

Table 15   Linear discriminant analysis: Variable Set II

Assessment no.	Percentage correct classification				No. patients
	Home	Part III	Continuing Care	Total	
1	66.7	60.0	84.6	69.5	59
2	61.1	40.0	76.9	61.0	59
3	85.7	100.0	80.0	86.1	36
4	88.9	100.0	100.0	94.7	19
5	100.0	100.0	100.0	100.0	12
6	100.0	100.0	100.0	100.0	8
7	100.0	50.0	100.0	75.0	4

Table 16   Linear discriminant analysis: Variable Set III

Assessment no.	Percentage correct classification				No. patients
	Home	Part III	Continuing Care	Total	
1	72.2	0.0	1.5	57.6	59
2	77.8	40.0	23.1	59.3	59
3	71.4	40.0	10.0	50.0	3619
4	33.3	50.0	66.7	47.4	12
5	14.3	33.3	100.0	33.3	8
6	0.0	66.7	100.0	37.5	4
7	100.0	50.0	100.0	75.0	

Table 17   Linear discriminant analysis: Variable Set IV

| Assessment no. | Percentage correct classification | | | | No. patients |
	Home	Part III	Continuing Care	Total	
1	58.3	10.0	53.8	49.2	59
2	63.9	10.0	46.2	50.8	59
3	71.4	20.0	50.0	58.3	36
4	77.8	50.0	66.7	68.4	19
5	0.0	33.3	50.0	16.7	12
6	0.0	33.3	100.0	25.0	8
7	100.0	0.0	100.0	50.0	4

study were admitted to the rehabilitation unit from other hospitals where, it may be surmised, they had been for varying lengths of time. It is possible, therefore, and quite likely, that the present study included more acutely ill patients who would simply not have been admitted to Stewart's rehabilitation unit and whose low scoring simply reflected the stage reached in their rehabilitation career.

Differences in samples are also implicated in the fact that 54 per cent of the present study sample returned to their home, compared with 20 per cent in Stewart's study and only 30 per cent went on to receive Continuing Care compared with 52 per cent in Stewart's study. The difference in percentages going home or on to Continuing Care may also indicate varying degrees of Social Services provision and differential pressure on hospital beds in the two areas.

Whatever the reasons for the failure to replicate, it is clear that for patients in the present study it is not possible to use the ADL score in order to predict progress. Only a crude distinction was seen on admission between the Home and Continuing Care groups, and on discharge between the Continuing Care group and both other groups. The lack of any statistically significant difference between the ADL scores of the Home and Part III groups probably reflects the degree of independence required for admission to a Part III home and the fact that social support as well as physical independence play a part in achieving a home discharge. In the present study one woman who scored zero was discharged to her home in the care of two sons without whom she would certainly have needed Continuing Care.

If prediction is to play any significant role, it must be employed at an early stage in the patient's stay in hospital, otherwise it loses its utility value in deployment of scarce resources. In this regard, mental status may have a role to play. It seems that those patients who scored 12 or more on admission, made progress and went home. However, it cannot be assumed that patients who do not score highly on admission will not make progress. Indeed, a transient confusional state may impair their performance at this stage, but, once the cause has been treated, e.g. antibiotics for a urinary tract infection, mental clarity may be restored and progress follow. It thus becomes crucial to determine the nature of mental confusion as early as possible and to distinguish between the dementia, the depression, and the toxic confusional state as these will have varying implications for the success of any rehabilitation programme.

In conclusion, it has not been possible to replicate Stewart's findings and it has not been possible to determine by means of an ADL assessment, those patients who will make progress. A high mental test score on admission to hospital indicates a likelihood of making progress, but a poor mental test score, depending on the cause, need not rule out the possibility of making progress. As most patients who were going to improve, did so within the first two weeks of their entry to the study, it is probably sensible to assume progress on behalf of all patients and combine this assumption with careful assessment of mental status and close monitoring of functional performance. In this way, no patients will miss their chance of making progress, but resources will not be expended wastefully when there is no indication of benefit.

References

Allen, C. M. C. (1984a). Predicting recovery after acute stroke, *Brit. J. Hosp. Med.*, **31** (6), 428–434.

Allen, C. M. C. (1984b). Predicting the outcome of acute stroke: a prognostic score. *J. Neurology, Neurosurgery, and Psychiatry*, **47**, 475–480.

Adler, M. K., Brown, C. C. and Acton, P. (1980). Stroke rehabilitation — is age a determinant? *J. Amer. Geriat. Soc.*, **28** (11), 499–503.

Brocklehurst, J. C., Andrews, K., Richards, B. and Laycock, P. J. (1978). How much physical therapy for patients with stroke? *B.M.J.*, **1**, 1307–1310.

Bruell, J. H. and Simon, J. I. (1960). Development of objective predictors of recovery in hemiplegic patients. *Arch. Phys. Med.*, **41**, 564–569.

Carroll, D. (1968). Qualitative assessment of physical disability, in P. J. R. Nicholls (Ed.), *Proceedings of a Symposium on the Motivation of the Physically Disabled*, pp. 48–56.

Denham, M. J. and Jeffreys, P. M. (1972). Routine mental teszing in the elderly. *Mod. Geriat.*, **2**, 75.

Dinnerstein, A. J., Lowenthal, M. and Dexter, M. (1965). Evaluation of a rating scale of ability in activities of daily living. *Arch. Phys. Med. Rehabil.*, Aug., 579–584.

Granger, C. V. Albrecht, G. L. and Hamilton, B. B. (1979). Outcome of comprehensive medical rehabilitation: measurement by PULSES profile and Barthel Index. *Arch. Phys. Med. Rehab.*, **60**, 141–154.

Hall, M. R. (1976). The assessment of disability in the geriatric patient. *Rheumatol, and Rehabil.*, **15** (2), 59–64.

Kahn, R. L. and Goldberg, A. I. (1960). The relationship of mental and physical status in institutionalised aged persons. *Amer. J. Psychiat.*, **117**, 120–124.

Katz, S., Downs, T. D., Cash, H. R. and Grotz R. C. (1970). Progress in development of the Index of ADL. *Gerontologist*, **10**, 20–30.

Lawton, M. P. and Brody, E. M. (1969). Assessment of older people: self-maintaining and instrumental activities of daily living. *Gerontologist*, **9**, 179–186.

Mahoney, F. I. and Barthel, D. W. (1965). Functional evaluation: the Barthel Index. *Rehabil.*, Feb., 61–65.

Peszczynski, M. (1961). Prognosis for rehabilitation of the older adult and the aged hemiplegic patient. *Amer. J. Cardiol.*, **7**, 365–369.

Pfeiffer, E. (Ed.) (1976). *Multidimensional Functional Assessment: The OARS Methodology*. A Manual. Durham, NC, Duke University Center for the Study of Aging.

Prescott, R. J. Garraway, W. M. and Akhtar, A. J. (1982). Predicting functional outcome following acute stroke using a standard clinical examination. *Stroke*, **13** (5), 641–647.

Qureshi, K. N. and Hodkinson, H. M. (1974). Evaluation of a ten question mental test in institutionalised Elderly. *Age and Ageing*, **3**, 152–157.

Roth, M. and Hopkins, B. (1953). Psychological test performance in patients over 60. *J. Ment. Sci.*, **99**, 439–450.

Sheikh, K. Smith, D. S., Meade, T. W., Goldenberg, E., Brennan, P. J. and Kinsella, G. (1979). Repeatability and validity of a modified activities of daily living (ADL) index in studies of chronic disability. *Int. Rehab. Med.*, **1**, 51–58.

Stewart, C. P. U. (1980). A prediction score for geriatric rehabilitation prospects. *Rheum. Rehabil.*, **19**, 239–245.

Wade, D. T., Skilbeck, C. E. and Hewer, R. L. (1983). Predicting Barthel ADL score at six months after an acute stroke. *Arch. Phys. Med. Rehabil.*, **64**, 24.

Appendix: Stewart's ADL Assessment Scale

ADL	Explanation of independence score	Score
Bowel	Faecal incontinence includes complete loss of bowel control and occasional soiling	0
	Complete control	15
Bladder + catheter	Urinary incontinence	0
	Dry by day or catheter dry	10
	Complete control	15
Walking + aid	Requires at least two nurses	0
	Walks with one nurse or an aid	10
	Complete independence safely	15

Dressing/undressing	Requires complete help	0
	Requires limited help (laces/zips)	5
	Dresses independently	10
On/off toilet	Requires help	0
	Independent safely	10
Feeding	Requires feeding	0
	Independent or including those who require food preparation	10
Wheelchair (only those unable to walk)	Unable to control safely	0
	Complete control	15
Stairs	Unsafe	0
	Able to climb five stairs safely	5
MSQ	Mental Status Questionnaire: two points per correct answer	0–20

Research in the Nursing Care of Elderly People
Edited by P. Fielding
© 1987 John Wiley & Sons Ltd

CHAPTER 7

Reliability and Validity of an In-patient Mobility Rating Scale

PAULINE FIELDING and
JANE FOSTER

Introduction

Various scales have been devised to measure a patient's physical capabilities, the latter being referred to as activities of daily living (ADL), rehabilitation, functional ability, self-care skills, functional capacity and motor activity, depending on how comprehensive are the physical capabilities referred to and in what circumstances the scales are used.

The uses of such scales are wide ranging. They sometimes describe the patient's present condition giving an indication of nursing requirements (Quigley, 1981); they can be used for goal setting and monitoring of progress (Klein and Bell, 1982; Jette, 1980); to provide a means of communication between staff caring for the patient (Donaldson, Wagner and Gresham, 1973); as an aid in discharge planning (Quigley, 1981); to teach staff and family members (Klein and Bell, 1982) and to provide a means of comparing clinical observations in rehabilitation research (Donaldson, Wagner and Gresham, 1973; Stewart, 1980).

Criteria for Scale Design

Validity

A scale should be valid, i.e. it should measure what it purports to measure (Liang and Jette, 1981). Bombardier and Tugwell (1982) distinguish the following kinds of validity with regard to the indices to be used in clinical trials.

Content validity — Is the choice of, and relative importance given to each component of the index appropriate for the purpose?

Face validity — Does the method of aggregating individual components into an index appear sensible?

Criterion validity — Does the index produce results that reflect the true clinical status of the patient?

Discriminant validity — Does the index detect the smallest improvement that is important?

Construct validity — Does the index agree with the expected results based on the hypothesis of the investigator?

Reliability

Functional assessment measures should also be reliable. Klein and Bell (1982) cite reliability as one of the basic qualities of an ADL scale, i.e. the scale should yield a reliable measure of a patient's current level of functioning. The use of such arbitrary verbal values as 'maximal' or 'minimal' to describe the amount of assistance required by a patient reduces inter-rater reliability. Raters will often differ in their opinions of exactly what constitutes 'maximal' or 'minimal'.

Downs and Fitzpatrick (1976) point to the same problem arising when nurses rely on subjective observations in their evaluations of an individual's health status. They claim that a nurse's observations vary according to her experiences and orientation. For this reason, among others, they chose a symbolic method of assessing body position and motor activity. Inter-rater reliability, therefore is threatened unless the assessment tool used overcomes the problem of observer bias.

The issue of intra-observer reliability is rather more vexed and can only be properly tested when one is sure that the level of function being assessed remains constant. This is clearly not the case when assessing patients at timed intervals when the purpose of the assessment is to detect changes in function.

Ease of Administration

The scale should be administratively practical. Hoberman, Cicenia and Stephenson (1952) suggest that it should be capable of use with bed, wheelchair or ambulant patients. Burton and Wright (1983) state that present measures of function are inclined to be too lengthy, too complex, and suffer from cross-cultural difficulties. The latter seems to refer to those measures requiring the patient to reply to questions regarding his functional capacity. It indicates that questions may be construed in different ways by people of different cultures thus causing a threat to the validity of the assessment.

The functional index must, therefore, be easy to use and understand; it should take a short time to complete, thus avoiding long, complicated activities which may tire the patient and themselves affect performance; and it should concentrate on the needs of particular groups of patients to avoid over-generalization.

Quantification

The scale should be easy to score and interpret and should allow quantification. Schoening *et al.* (1965) describe how early rehabilitators found that a straightforward description of the activities of daily living was a simple and concrete means of measuring functional capacity. Such descriptions were easy to complete, and demonstrated progress towards treatment goals.

However, their value was limited when the clinician wanted to look at the progress of a group of patients, as there was no quantification of the relative value of individual activities of daily living, or of the total functional capacity of the patient. In most assessments of the activities of daily living, the ability to walk is not differentiated quantitatively from the ability to brush one's teeth independently, yet the former is more important in regard to total physical independence. Schoening and his colleagues see quantification, therefore, as a means of assessing the progress of a group of patients and also the total functional capacity of a patient.

Liang and Jette (1981) point out, however, that quantification is also vital to the ability to evaluate the effectiveness of an intervention, to help in defining the need for specific services or therapy and to monitor the longitudinal course of a disease. They warn that individuals differ in their perception of what is important when weighting items in a scale and that statistically sound instruments may produce results devoid of clinical meaning or significance. The aim should be then, to produce a system of measurement that is simple yet comprehensive and with mathematical properties that allow the manipulation of the data to produce clinically interpretable results.

Specification of Circumstances

Dunt *et al.* (1980) emphasize the importance of specifying the circumstances under which ADLs are performed, whether with physical aids or adaptations, or with personal assistance as these can affect performance to a varying and unknown extent. They recommend differential measurement according to the circumstances, suggesting that measurement without aids or adaptations and assistance is most appropriate in incidence or prevalence studies of chronic diseases and in outcome studies of the effect of biomedical care. They go on to suggest that measurement of performance with aids or adaptations is most appropriate in studies of independence whilst the introduction of assistance will be relevant when the total impact of all caring services is being assessed. Therefore, researchers should specify the circumstances under which the scale is used in order to produce reliable and unambiguous results.

Problems of Scale Design

Inappropriate Design

Assessment scales can be used for different purposes and with different types of patient. The latter may be young people recovering from the effects of trauma, elderly people recovering from the effects of stroke or people of any age suffering from chronic disease such as rheumatoid arthritis. Expectations of recovery may be certain, possible or impossible. The object of using the scale may be to assess the amount of care required, to monitor progress or deterioration or to assess treatment needed. The scale may be required to cover all activities of daily living or a selected few. Bombardier and Tugwell (1982) warn that because of the widely varying purposes for which they are used an index that has been developed for one purpose may be quite unsuitable for another.

Extent of Functional Capacity

Liang and Jette (1981) point out that functional capacity is relative to the patient's expectations, priorities, goals and social support. These can result in different patients reacting differently to apparently similar levels of physical impairment.

Classification and Measurement

Burton and Wright (1983) note that it may be difficult to judge the importance of things which patients can do with or without aids. The patient's perception of what is important or even essential may be very different from that of the carer. Similarly, not all items of function will be measurable. Liang and Jette (1982) point out that easily measured items which comprise scales that are ideal for statistical manipulation may bear questionable relation to functional ability.

Problems of Assessment Scales

Global Statements

Klein and Bell (1982) claim that previous ADL scales sometimes stated items too globally. In this way the individual components which make up each item are ignored. Failure to consider any one specific component may result in the observer missing a clue to the nature of a problem. Global items are thus insensitive to slight changes in functioning. Klein and Bell also suggest that some scales embrace too many aspects of functioning, e.g. ADL function combined with mental status to yield a single score, the units of which differ widely.

Arbitrary Verbal Values

Some scales use values such as 'maximal' or 'moderate' which may not have a common meaning to all people. Klein and Bell (1982) suggest that where such values are used there is a reduction in inter-rater reliability.

Interpretation of Total Scores

The interpretation of a total score which combines many different categories can be problematic. For example on a ten-item scale with a four-point rating, a total of 20 may mean that equal, moderate assistance is needed on all items or that there is complete dependence on five items and complete independence on the remainder. In order to interpret the meaning of the scale it will be necessary to examine individual item scores as well as the total score.

Timed Performances

Timing the length of performance of any particular function may affect the validity of the scale. Timing is irrelevant if the function cannot be performed and timing may be more or less important in different settings.

Methods of Assessment

Most authors have measured a number of activities of daily living on a nominal dependence scale of 0–4 or 5. However, the number items included and the detail therein varies considerably.

Parish and James (1982) assessed twenty items simply recording whether the patient was 'dependent' or 'independent' for each item. As each item subsumed a number of functions there was no scope for pinpointing specific areas of difficulty, e.g. 'Transfer' was described as, 'Move out of bed/chair onto feet and sit/lie down after standing (or into/out of a wheelchair if wheelchair mobile).'

By contrast, Dinnerstein, Lowenthal and Dexter (1965) devised a scale which allowed for more precision in assessment. They identified eleven areas of functioning which were scored on a 0–5 nominal scale. Each of the eleven areas were subdivided into six items, breaking the function down into more discrete items as in the following extract:

'Transfer from bed'
1. Roll to side
2. Feet from covers over edge
3. Come to sitting at edge
4. Maintain sitting balance
5. Prepare for transfer
6. Transfer
(Dinnerstein, Lowenthal and Dexter, 1965)

Jette (1980) rated non-institutionalized arthritic patients not only on their level of dependence but also on pain and difficulty. His aim was to assess functional capacity in order to judge the effectiveness of care. Each of 45 items were rated on dependence, pain and difficulty scales and he suggests that the resulting 135 separate pieces of data for each assessment might be successfully reduced by more than half if only two items from each of the five major functional categories are chosen. The category of physical mobility accounted for the largest proportion of the variance (16.1 per cent) in the dependence scores.

Sheikh *et al.* (1980) also describe a method of assessment which tests patients in more than one dimension. This method, which is for the assessment of motor function in patients with chronic disability, scores patients on both affected limb and total body function. Unlike other scales mentioned here, independence is not measured. Limb and body movement is not applied to the context of daily living.

Downs and Fitzpatrick (1976) also studied actual body movement but related this to activities of daily living. Their aim was to evaluate the health status of patients whose physical abilities were limited in some way. It does not appear that their assessment was aimed at any particular group of patients or type of disability.

They rated patients at 15-second intervals as follows:

1 Body Position
   (a) Upright
   (b) Sitting
   (c) Lying down
   (d) Leaning
   (e) Leaning over
   (f) Kneeling

2 Body Movement
   (a) Head active
   (b) Right leg active
   (c) Left leg active
   (d) Both legs active
   (e) Right arm active
   (f) Left arm active
   (g) Both arms active
   (h) Both arms and legs active

Body movement was then classified as 'minimal', 'moderate' or 'high' in intensity of activity. Each body position, movement and intensity rating was noted by symbols marked on a chart at 15-second intervals over a period of five minutes, thus, twenty evaluations in each of three categories were made.

Problems in assessment by this method arose in patients who exhibited constant action and in patients who demonstrated more complex movements, the latter resulting in low inter-rater reliability.

The scale which is the subject of this study was developed by Susan Kilford (personal communication) in order to provide a measure of the 'basic mobility skills' of hospital in-patients. Kilford hoped that this scale would relate to the amount of nursing intervention required, thus helping nurses to organize their work more effectively and to communicate information about patients more accurately. The scale appears in full in the appendix to this chapter.

Method

Sample

The sample was drawn from a population of elderly women under the care of a geriatrician in an acute geriatric ward, who were described by the nursing staff as having some problem in mobilizing. Patients who were demented or deemed too poorly to participate, were excluded. $n = 21$ Age range $= 74$–89 years   Mean age $= 80$ years.

Instrument

Kilford's In-patient Mobility Scale.

Procedure

In each case, the patient was fully informed, by the researcher, of the nature of the study, its purpose, and her role in it. Where possible, a written consent was also obtained.

   Patients were selected to take part in the study as soon after their admission as possible. Their degree of mobility was rated simultaneously but independently by the researcher and by a trained nurse on the ward. A separate written evaluation of the patient's mobility was also elicited from the nurse who was caring for the patient on that shift. In this way the following were obtained:

(a) A measure of inter-rater reliability
(b) A measure of discriminant validity.

If the patient remained on the ward for more than one week the ratings were repeated at weekly intervals. Thus a total of 41 evaluations were obtained.

Results

Inter-rater Reliability

Percentage agreement between raters on the total scores for each patient varied from 42.9 – 100 per cent agreement. No relationship could be found between the patients' total scores on the scales and the percentage agreement between raters. In other words, no particular level of mobility appeared to result in a higher or lower percentage agreement than any other. The overall inter-rater reliability was 76.6 per cent. Table 1 shows that percentage agreement also varied considerably between the different items on the scale, with chair activities presenting the most problems.

Table 1   Inter-rater reliability and individual items

Item	% Agreement
Getting up from chair	53.7
Sitting down in chair	63.4
Getting out of bed	70.7
Getting into bed	70.7
Walking to bathroom toilet and back	90.2
Walking short distance	90.2

Discriminant Validity

The written evaluations of mobility were examined for mention of the same items which were included in the scale and for mention of other items which were not included in the scale. The number of scale items mentioned ranged from 1–5 per nurse with a mean of 2.8 items. Mentions of non-scale items ranged from 1–6 per nurse with a mean of 2.9 items. Using Spearman's rank correlation coefficient, a positive correlation was found between the number of mentions of scale and non-scale items ($r_s = 0.3$ d.f. 39 Significant at 5 per cent level).

Table 2 shows those non-scale items most frequently mentioned by nurses. Patients' feelings about mobilizing included the patient's level of confidence or lack of it; the security gained from the use of a frame or from holding someone's arm, anxiety, nervousness or agitation generated by having to move and the general level of awareness of capability. Balance, which accounted for nine mentions covered the ability to stand without support and the maintenance of stability. The patient's ability to use the toilet and/or bath was clearly important to many nurses. It included the ability to get on and off the toilet, into and out of the bath, the need for help with the adjustment of clothing or pads and the ability to negotiate the toilet door. Nurses also mentioned the type of walking aid used and whether or not the patient used it properly. If there was a clinical condition present which affected leg movement, then this was also mentioned, as was the manner in which the patient walked, e.g. very slowly.

Table 2   Non-scale items and frequency of mention

Item	No. mentions
Patient's feeling about mobilizing	15
Dyspnoea	9
Balance	9
Ability to us toilet/bath	7
Type of aid use and effectiveness	7
Disease affecting leg movement	6
Manner of working	6

Other non-scale items which were mentioned by one or two nurses only included the patient's need for encouragement to mobilize; the limiting factor of poor eyesight, tiredness and pain; the distance the patient was able to walk; movement in bed as a preparation to getting out of bed; idiosyncrasies of movement and orientation in time and place.

Discussion

Inter-rater Reliability

Overall, the level of inter-rater reliability contained too much variance for the scale to be useful without further modification. The results indicate that the more complicated tasks resulted in a lower percentage agreement between raters. For example, getting up from a chair involves several discrete movements for an elderly person with problems of mobility. These may include the following:

(a) Placing frame or sticks in a convenient position.
(b) Moving to the edge of seat.

(c) Placing feet flat on floor in correct position.
(d) Placing hands on arm-rest or convenient support.
(e) Leaning forward.
(f) Pushing down on arms of chair.
(g) Lifting up and taking weight on feet.
(h) Transferring hands to frame or sticks.
(i) Maintaining balance and stability.

Once the patient is standing upright it is then a much easier task to evaluate their mobility score for walking a short distance. given the wide range of inter-rater reliability it would be very important to use the same rater each time if the scale were used to monitor a patient's progress.

Discriminant Validity

Experience in using the scale and comparison with written mobility evaluations, has illustrated several weaknesses on the part of the scale. The scale omits any mention of the patient's mobility in bed. This is important not only with regard to dependency but as a prelude to getting out of bed. The criteria regarding walking to the bathroom/toilet and back do not include any mention of the patient needing assistance with clothing or the changing of incontinence pads. These are surely important items for inclusion as the knowledge that a patient can walk to the toilet or bathroom and back is of little value with regard to the nursing care required if a nurse has to assist the patient once he or she is in the bathroom or toilet. This is perhaps an instance where mobility is being artificially separated from an activity of daily living and in the process being rendered somewhat irrelevant in isolation. The 'activity' of going to the bathroom/toilet may include at least the following:

(a) Getting on and off the toilet.
(b) Arranging clothes/changing pads.
(c) Manipulating hot and cold taps safely.

Knowing that the patient can travel there and back simply does not convey sufficient information for the nurse to assess the level of help required. It is clear from the results that discriminant validity of the scale is not high and consequently the scale will need further modification to include those items noted by nurses as being important factors affecting mobility.

During the data collection period, two other factors were noted which threatened the validity of the scale. Firstly, the distance between bed and toilet — the scale did not show up the fact that one patient, between assessments, had become very dyspnoeic and consequently her bed had been moved nearer to the toilet. Therefore, although she scored '2' on the first assessment, when she walked the length of the ward and back with comparative ease, on the second assessment she still scored '2' for walking a few metres to the toilet which she did with difficulty. If this patient were to have been transferred to another ward, there would have been no clue from the mobility scale that her level of mobility had decreased, nor that she needed to have a bed close to the toilet if she were to be able to walk there.

Secondly, it was noted that the patient's mobility could be influenced by the type of shoes or slippers she was wearing. If slippers were soft, with sides and backs which did not easily return to an upright supportive position when the patient had put them on, they could make it difficult for the patient to get into a standing position, and of course were dangerous to walk in. Slippers were also seen to be difficult for patients to kick off when getting into bed. Few of the patients were able to reach down with their hands to remove or put on their slippers. Therefore, a patient's level on the mobility scale, and their subsequent nursing needs, could be affected by the provision of shoes or slippers which have a degree of stiffness, are easy to put on and which stay on securely as the patient walks.

Two factors which directly influence mobility and yet are not included in the scale are mental status and eyesight. Many hospitalized elderly patients may be temporarily disoriented in time and place. Such patients, no matter how adept at mobilizing, would always need nursing supervision in order to ensure their own and others' safety. Likewise, an indication of poor eyesight would alert nurses to the possibility of an otherwise safely mobile patient injuring themselves if objects were in their path.

General Problems in the use of a Mobility Scale

Adopting the use of a scale to measure a patient's mobility means overcoming several problems which, if ignored, could threaten the validity of the assessment.

Firstly, staff must be trained in the use of a scale and this, depending on the other activity in the clinical setting, and the speed of staff turnover, may be more or less problematic. Facility in using a scale involves not only applying the details of the criteria attached to each item but, from the nurse's point of view, resisting the temptation to help until it is quite clear that the optimum level of performance has been achieved.

Secondly, co-operation on the part of the patient must be secured. Some patients in the present study, who agreed to take part when it was explained to them, subsequently declined saying that they were too tired or simply did not wish to be bothered. Changes in mood or tiredness bring about alterations in motivation to co-operate in an assessment. The scale does not allow for the fact that although a patient could achieve a given score on one occasion, on another a similar level of performance may require a great deal more persuasion and encouragement.

Advantages in the use of a Mobility Scale

Use of a mobility scale ensures that an assessment, and thus a record is made of performance on certain items. When nurses were asked to provide a written evaluation of their patient's mobility, they covered an average of 5.7 items in all. Therefore, the use of the present scale which consists of six items ensures a more thorough assessment than would otherwise take place.

The use of a mobility scale highlights deficits as well as achievements in performance. Written assessments tended to focus only on what the patient could do and gave little or no attention to items which could not be performed. Nurses were not, it seemed, selecting from a large range of mobility items and considering the patient's performance in any systematic way. Rather, they were providing a highly individualized picture of one particular patient's capabilities in respect of a fairly narrow aspect of mobility. There is clearly a need for nurses to employ a more systematic and structured approach to the assessment of mobility, whilst retaining their ability to individualize patients' problems.

In conclusion, inter-rater reliability was not high in this study. Modification of more complex items may improve reliability. Discriminant validity was not sufficiently comprehensive and could probably be improved by further expansion of the scale to include relevant items. However, using the mobility assessment scale ensured a more complete assessment of the patient's mobility than did nurses' written evaluations alone. Future work should be directed towards producing a more comprehensive scale for nurses to use which will embrace those non-scale items highlighted in this study as having relevance for mobility.

References

Burton, K. E. and Wright, V. (1983). Functional assessment. *Br. J. Rheum.*, **22** Supplement, 44–47.

Bombardier, C. and Tugwell, P. (1982). A methodological framework to develop and select indices for clinical trials: statistical and judgmental approach. *J. Rheum.*, 753–774.

Dinnerstein, A. J., Lowenthal, M. and Dexter, M. (1965). Evaluation of a rating scale of ability in activities of daily living. *Arch. Phys. Med. Rehabil.*, Aug., 579–584.

Donaldson, S. W., Wagner, C. C. and Gresham, G. E. (1973). *Arch. Phys. Med. Rehabil.*, **54**, 175–179.

Downs, F. and Fitzpatrick, J. (1976). Preliminary investigation of the reliability and validity of a tool for the assessment of body position and motor activity. *Nursing Research*, Nov-Dec., **25**, 6.

Dunt, D. R., Kaufert, J. M., Corkhill, R., Creese, A. L., Green, S. and Locker, D. (1980). A technique for precisely measuring activities of daily living. *Community Medicine*, **2**, 120–125.

Hoberman, M., Cicenia, E. F. and Stephenson, G. R. (1952). Daily activity testing in physical therapy and rehabilitation. *Arch. Phys. Med.*, Feb., 99–108.

Jette, A. M. (1980). Functional capacity evaluation: an empirical approach. *Arch. Phys. Med. Rehab.*, **61**, 85–89.

Kilford, S. (personal communication).

Klein, R. and Bell, P. (1982). Self-care skills. Behavioural measurement with Klein–Bell ADL-Scale. *Arch. Phys. Med. Rehab.*, **63**, 235–238.

Liang, M. H. and Jette, H. M. (1981). Measuring functional ability in chronic arthritis. *Arthritis and Rheumatism*, **24**, 1, 80–86.

Parish, J. G. and James, D. W. (1982). A method for evaluating the level of independence during the rehabilitation of the disabled. *Rheumatol. Rehabil.*, **21**, 107–114.

Quigley, P. A., (1981). Nursing evaluation in rehabilitation. *Rehabilitation Nursing*, Nov–Dec., 12–14.

Schoening, H. A., Anderigg, L., Bergstrom, D., Fonda, M., Steinke, N. and Ulrich, P. (1965). Numerical scoring of self-care status of patients. *Arch. Phys. Med. Rehabil.*, **46**, 689–698.

Sheikh, K., Smith, D. S., Meade, T. W., Brennan, P. J. and Ide, O. (1980). Assessment of motor function in studies of chronic disability, *Rheumatol. Rehabil.* **19**, 83–90.

Stewart, C. P. U. (1980). A prediction score for geriatric rehabilitation prospects, *Rheum. Rehab.*, **19**, 239–245.

Appendix: Kilford's Inpatient Mobility Rating Scale

Activities:

1. Getting out of bed.
   This includes the patient being able to achieve a sitting position on the edge of the bed and putting on shoes or slippers.
2. Getting into bed.
   This includes the patient being able to remove shoes or slippers before getting into bed.
3. Getting up from a chair.
4. Sitting down in a chair.
   Both these items require the use of the patient's usual chair.
5. Walking to bathroom/toilet and back.
   This includes opening and closing toilet door.
6. Walking short distance.
   This is defined as 2–3 metres around bed area.

Score: Each item is scored on a six point scale, 0–5 as follows.

   0 = Completely independent and safe
   1 = Unaided, but has some difficulty
   2 = Uses mechanical aid and/or adapted equipment
   3 = Needs help/supervision from nurse
   4 = Needs help from two nurses
   5 = Does not perform activity even with help

Note: It should be noted that Kilford originally included a seventh activity (stair climbing and descending) which has not been included here because of its lack of relevance to the particular sample of patients.

Research in the Nursing Care of Elderly People
Edited by P. Fielding
Published by John Wiley & Sons Ltd
© Crown Copyright 1987

CHAPTER 8

A Study of Non-verbal Communication Between Nurses and Elderly Patients

ANDRÉE C. LE MAY and SALLY J. REDFERN

This century has seen a marked increase in the number of people aged over 65 living in the United Kingdom. In 1983 the elderly formed 15 per cent (8.4 m) of the population, with 41 per cent (3.4 m) of this group aged over 75 years ('old' elderly). By the year 2000 the increase in the 'old' elderly will be substantial and will be accompanied by a proportional reduction in those people aged between 65 and 74 years ('young' elderly) (OPCS, 1983).

The large numbers of very old people in the population, and the projected change in the composition of this group has important implications for nurses and nursing. With an increase in dependency and disability with age, it is old people particularly who need nursing care. Although informal carers provide most of the care (Evers, 1986), the rising number of very old people proportional to 'young' elderly, together with family mobility and more women in paid employment outside the home, means that the family will find it increasingly difficult to meet the needs of their frail elders. Many of the carers are spouses and children who are pensioners themselves, and their own health and vigour may be failing. Nurses in all settings, except paediatric and maternity units, can expect old people to make up an increasing proportion of their client group.

Elderly people have survived most of this century and have lived through experiences very different from those of their nurses (severe Victorian values, two world wars, depression and austerity, etc.). These old survivors are likely to hold attitudes and values based on experiences which contrast markedly with those of young nurses. It follows

171

that the gap of one, or more likely, two generations which separate elderly patients from their nurses makes effective communication between them difficult. Nurses need particular skill in communicating with old people in a way which conveys a sensitive and caring attitude but which is not cloying nor patronizing.

This chapter highlights the non-verbal element of nurse–patient communication. First we define non-verbal communication and list its main components. We continue with a review of the literature associated with one of these components, touch. The second part of the chapter focuses on our research concerning the nature and frequency of nurse–patient touch, and its relationship to the physical and psychological well-being of elderly patients.

Non-verbal Communication

What is Non-verbal Communication?

Non-verbal communication is simply a way of describing all behaviours which transmit messages without the use of a verbal language. It is an important form of communication which can convey messages between communicators by itself, or in conjunction with a verbal language. Non-verbal communication can be divided into two categories — vocal non-verbal communication and non-vocal non-verbal communication. Mehrabian (1972) estimated that 38 per cent of meaning was transmitted by vocal non-verbal communication, 55 per cent by non-vocal non-verbal communication and 7 per cent by words.

If we look at the components of each category we can see how complex the non-verbal communication system is.

Vocal non-verbal communication, or 'paralanguage', consists of all the non-verbal accompaniments of words, for example pitch, intonation, speech rate, volume, fluency and dialect. These cues make our voices unique, allow us to emphasize important words, convey our feelings and moods and in the case of dialect, allow us to glimpse the communicator's origins. In addition to these voice qualities there are other non-verbal sounds that enhance the meaning of the communication. These include laughter, crying, groans, yawns and vocalized hesitations (ums, ers, ahs, etc.).

The non-vocal element of non-verbal communication includes: body movement (posture, gesture, facial expression and eye behaviour), physical appearance, timing of communications, personal space and territoriality and touch. All five categories are important in the transmission of feelings, emotional states, personality and attitudes. In this chapter, we are primarily interested in the last category, touch.

Touch — the Literature

An Introduction

Touching is a highly potent way of communicating with another person. Touch has been defined by Watson (1975, p. 104) as 'an intentional physical contact between two or more individuals'. Watson divides touch into two categories: 'Instrumental touch', which is a deliberate physical contact necessary to perform a task, e.g. taking a pulse, or giving a bed bath and 'expressive touch', which is relatively spontaneous and affective, and is not necessary for the completion of a task, e.g. hand-holding or an arm around the shoulder.

Touch has been described as a basic human need, which the foetus may respond to from as early as eight weeks gestation (Montagu, 1971). Throughout infancy touch continues to be important, fostering love, gratification, closeness and comfort as well as being a primary form of communication, orientation and learning. But despite its importance, as the child grows older (s)he becomes less dependent on touch as a necessary link with his or her environment and is influenced by the social mores and taboos associated with touching. She/he may learn to limit the use of touch to special occasions, permitted shows of affection or for comfort. Suddenly touching has become risky and open to misinterpretation by others.

Despite the restrictions we place on touching it continues to be important for most of us throughout adulthood. The need for touch does not disappear with age and maturity. Bowlby (1958) suggests that although non-intimate touch tends not to be as frequent between adults compared with adult–child touch, the frequency which was common in childhood can recur in situations of danger, incapacity and sickness. This suggests that becoming a patient may lead to an increased need for touch, a view also expressed by Dominian (1971), Barnett (1972a) and Goodykoontz (1979).

Touch and Nursing

As nurses we are in a unique and privileged position as far as touching patients is concerned. The unwritten rules about touch are relaxed somewhat in the nurse–patient relationship, and both nurses and patients give and accept touches which they would regard as unthinkable outside sickness. Touching is an integral part of nursing, which, if used wisely should become a fundamental and vital component of communication. Barnett (1972a) identifies groups of patients who may benefit particularly from communication through touch, such as patients with an altered body image, those who feel depersonalized, or are dependent or anxious, or have a lowered self-esteem or are dying.

Touching facilitates nurse–patient interactions, it promotes health and well-being and indicates the concern, interest and care that nurses have for patients (Goodykoontz, 1979). Touching can also help to reduce patients' anxiety. Goodykoontz suggests that many elderly people suffer from a change in body image associated with ageing, deformity or disability, and that touch by nurses can communicate acceptance and reassurance to them. Touch can be very powerful in conveying to a vulnerable person that (s)he is an important and valued individual.

A general lack of 'non-essential' touch between health team workers and patients was observed in a study by Barnett (1972b). She found that the amount of touch used varied within the hospital team with registered nurses and junior nursing students using more than senior nursing students and junior doctors. The nurses who most frequently used touch were aged between 18 and 25 years, and the patients most frequently touched were between 26 and 33 years. Patients aged between 6 and 17, and over 65 years received the least touch. These findings are supported by Goodykoontz (1979) and by Watson's (1975) suggestion that patients over 65 years are deprived of touch.

Other studies which used an evaluative research design have shown the importance of touch in different nursing specialities. In maternity wards, mothers who received appropriate and meaningful touch during labour and post-partum handled their infants more effectively than those receiving remote or impersonal touch (Rubin, 1963). Lorensen (1983) found that labour was shorter for primigravid women who received purposeful touch (stroking and affectionate hugs) compared with a group who received usual care. The touched women perceived the nurse as being helpful in relieving their discomfort during labour. Touch may therefore have a calming and comforting effect upon patients in pain, and it may be effective for all patients when in a crisis.

In the surgical area, Whitcher and Fisher (1979) carried out an experimental study to examine the effects on patients' psychological and physiological responses of nurses holding the patient's hand during preoperative teaching. They used a 2 (touch versus no touch) × 2 (male versus female) research design with a sample of patients awaiting elective surgery. Outcome measures were chosen to determine the patients' psychological and physiological response to touch. The results indicated that women in the touched group experienced more favourable reactions than men in both groups and than women in the no-touch group, i.e. lowered anxiety, more positive feelings towards the nurses who used touch together with more reciprocal touch, more preoperative teaching booklet reading and more favourable post-operative physiological responses (lower blood pressure). The authors suggest that the men's negative response stems from their socialization against showing dependency and discomfort. These findings support Watson's (1975) suggestion that men, except when under extreme stress, or the very old, are less accepting than women of non-sexual touch by women.

In coronary care and intensive care units, the effect of arm touching together with verbal interaction on patients' tenseness revealed more positive responses and less tenseness in the touched group (McCorkle, 1974). McCorkle concluded that touch increased the value of the communication by making the patients attentive, by perceiving the interaction as more meaningful and the nurse as being more interested in them and more caring.

The positive effects of touch have been highlighted by Aguilera (1967) who studied touch and verbal interaction between nurses and patients in psychiatric wards. Her findings suggest that touching by nurses increased the patients' verbal interaction, their rapport with others and their approach behaviour.

Despite these potentially positive effects of touch, authors emphasize the need for caution. Touch can be risky and nurses should recognize patients' needs for personal space and for privacy. Touch may even be contraindicated for certain individuals or on certain occasions (Barnett, 1972a). Touch may be misinterpreted by nurses or patients and it may increase anxiety if the recipient has a limited awareness of touch (De Augustinis, Sani and Kumler, 1963). Some nurses may have become so socialized against touch that they need to be shown its appropriateness before they are comfortable and effective in its use. Communicating in nursing is a skilled process and its components need to be taught.

Touch and Elderly People

The importance and effect of touch with the elderly has been examined by several authors. Burnside (1973) suggests that touch may help old people to decrease sensory deprivation, to increase reality orientation and to alleviate pain. In more recent work, Burnside (1981) draws our attention to practices nurses use which restrict touching. Examples are the use of geriatric chairs and wheelchairs which make it difficult to touch patients, and cot sides which isolate the patient from physical contact with others.

Watson (1975) studied the use of touch by nurses with severely impaired patients in a home for the elderly and noted certain factors that were important in the touching behaviours he observed. The body areas most likely to be touched were those furthest from the genital zone; patients and nurses of the same sex were more likely to touch each other; and more touch occurred with the less physically impaired patient. Watson also noted that more expressive touch was used by more senior nurses, which supports Henley (1973), suggesting that initiators of touch are often of a higher status than receivers of touch. Watson highlights the likelihood of touch deprivation in male and severely impaired patients.

Nurses can try to maintain contact with confused elderly patients by using more expressive touch, which may convey acceptance and empathy, as well as having a calming effect on patients and increasing the likelihood of communication (Seaman, 1982). The confused patient's use of and acceptance of touch should be included in the patient's care plan and communicated to others in the nursing team. In this way all the nurses would know the patient's preferences, and touch would become a recognized nursing intervention, and its effects evaluated.

Elderly patients perceive nurses who touch them as being ready to listen and help as well as liking them (Ernst and Shaw, 1980). Ernst and Shaw suggest that touch can decrease isolation, strengthen interactions, indicate caring and validate a patient's existence. For old people, the need for touch may be greater and may be a more effective mode of communication than the need to talk, particularly for those whose other senses are declining (Burton and Heller, 1964; Preston, 1973; Ernst and Shaw, 1980). An elderly person often relies on touch to gather information about the environment. Touch promotes trust, empathy, perceptual stimulation and enhances the effects of other forms of communication, particularly for this age group (Hollinger, 1980).

Copstead (1980) describes the frequency of touch between permanently institutionalized elderly patients and registered nurses, during medicine rounds, and the effects of the touch on patients' subsequent self-appraisal and interaction with nurses. Twenty-two of the 33 patients observed were touched, mainly on the wrist or hand. In this touched group nurse–patient interactions were longer, and patients had more positive self-appraisals than those in the not touched group. Copstead suggests that nurses can use touch to foster patients' self worth. She challenges nurses to use more meaningful touch during nursing procedures.

De Wever (1977) investigated 99 nursing-home patients' responses to nurses' expressive touch. She showed patients pictures of four different nurses (one male and one female in their early twenties and one male and one female in their early forties), and asked them how comfortable they would feel receiving specific touches, e.g. placing a hand on the patient's face, arm or around the shoulder, from each of the nurses photographed. The results led her to advise the judicious use of expressive touch because not all patients found nurses' touch comfortable. Men particularly were more likely than women to feel uncomfortable, especially if the nurse was male. De Wever suggests that a touch on the arm or face may be more acceptable to many elderly patients than an arm around the shoulder.

The effects of touch on communication with elderly confused patients and nurses were studied by Langland and Panicucci (1982). They used an experimental design and observed 32 elderly female nursing-home patients. In both experimental and control groups patients were asked to perform a particular action (taking a calendar from the nurse's tray), and the experimental group also received a light touch on the forearm from the nurse. Both groups' non-verbal (facial expressions, eye contact and body movement) and verbal responses were observed as well as their performance of the requested action. The results showed a significant increase in positive non-verbal responses of the touched group. Patients in the experimental group gave more verbal responses, and more of them attempted the task than the controls, but these differences were not significant. The authors recommend the deliberate use of touch by nurses, and suggest that touch may be important in reducing sensory deprivation in nursing-home patients.

In conclusion, the literature, which is mainly American, suggests that the appropriate use of touch by nurses may enhance patient well-being and comfort, particularly for those patients who may be deprived of much needed touch. The research in this area raises several questions about the use of touch by nurses:

— The frequency with which nurses use expressive touch in comparison to instrumental touch.

— The factors which affect nurses' use of touch and patients' acceptance of touch.
— The effect of touch on patients' moods, morale and well-being.
— The extent to which patients want to be touched, and whether nurses feel comfortable when touching.

The study described below has been designed in an attempt to answer these questions for elderly patients and their nurses.

The Study

A preliminary feasibility study (Porter *et al.*, 1986) confirmed that it was possible to record and classify touch as well as its associated variables (e.g. the nurse's and patient's position, and the task or nature of the interaction in which touch occurs). We were also able to identify individual differences which influence the use of or acceptance of touch (e.g. age, sex, patient's socio-economic status, grade of nurse, patient's diagnosis and degree of dependency), and to assess the patient's well-being.

This preliminary work gave us confidence to design a larger study, which at the time of writing (January 1986) is still in progress. It has the following aims:

1 To observe the amount and type of touch used by nurses caring for elderly people in different settings (e.g. acute geriatric, rehabilitation and long-term care wards, a day hospital and a private nursing home).
2 To identify individual characteristics of patients and nurses which affect the use and acceptance of touch.
3 To establish whether nurses' attitudes towards elderly people affect the amount and type of touch they use.
4 To determine whether patient dependency and well-being affect the use of touch by nurses.
5 To establish whether there is a relationship between touch and patient well-being.

The methods are based mainly on observation and interview techniques.

Method for Aim 1

Observation of touch is patient centred and occurs during the day shift for each selected consenting patient. Since nurse–patient touch, particularly instrumental touch, occurs very rapidly it is essential to record all the information relevant to each touch quickly and accurately. A touch observation schedule was designed (Porter *et al.*, 1986) and subsequently modified for this purpose (Figure 1).

The following components of each touch episode are recorded on the schedule:

(i) *When* the touch occurred in the nurse–patient interaction, that is during the approach, at the interface, or at separation from it.
(ii) *Duration* of the nurse–patient interaction, e.g. feeding, bathing, dressing.
(iii) *Length* of each touch episode within the nurse–patient interaction.
(iv) *Type of touch* — instrumental, expressive or indefinable.
(v) *Body area* touched.
(vi) *Response* of the recipient to the touch, that is:
(a) silence, verbal or non-verbal communication, (b) the nature of the verbal response (positive, neutral or negative), and (c) the type of non-verbal communication (e.g. crying, eye contact, laughter).
(vii) *Verbal communication* of the toucher and its nature (emotional/ psycho-social, treatment/care, social chat, or silence).
(viii) *The task* or nature of the interaction being performed.
(ix) *The patient's position* (e.g. lying, sitting, walking).
(x) *The nurse's position* (e.g. sitting, standing, walking).

Inter-observer Reliability

Inter-observer reliability of the touch observation schedule has so far been assessed on three occasions — once using videotapes of nurse–patient interactions, and twice in long-term care wards. This was done by calculating reliability coefficients (using the kappa coefficient (Cohen, 1960)) between two observers, each of whom independently observed and recorded the same nurse–patient interaction. A total of 546 touches were recorded during these sessions. However of these only 407 (75 per cent) were recorded by both observers and form the basis for the reliability calculations. The 139 (25 per cent) remaining touches were discarded as observers either recorded different episodes or only one observer had recorded the episode.

A kappa coefficient can range from −1 to +1 but one of $\geqslant 0.60$ has

Date ....
Place ....
Episode no ....
I.D. Code   N .... P ....

WHEN   NURSE / PATIENT
Approach ☐
Interface ☐
Separation ☐

Duration ....

Length ....

PATIENT / NURSE RESPONSE
Silence ☐

Verbal   Positive ☐
            Neutral ☐
            Negative ☐

Non-verbal ☐
Type ....

VERBAL COMMUNICATION
Emotional / Psyco-social ☐
Treatment / Care ☐
Social Chat ☐
Other ☐   Silence ☐

TASK ....
....

PATIENT POSITION   NURSE POSITION
Getting up / down ☐   Kneel / Squatting ☐
Standing ☐   Sitting bed ☐
Walking ☐   Sitting chair ☐
Lying ☐   Standing ☐
Sitting bed ☐   Walking ☐
Sitting chair ☐   Other ☐
Other ☐

RESEARCHER'S NOTES ....
....
....
....

Figure 1   The touch observation schedule

been suggested as indicating an acceptable level of reliability (Cichetti, 1984). A problem arises with the kappa coefficient when insufficient variability in the data occurs. Some of the components of the schedule were unsuitable for kappa calculations for this reason, and so percentage agreement was calculated. A percentage agreement of ≥ 70 was taken as an acceptable level.

Table 1   Inter-observer reliability of the components of the touch schedule

Component	Video		Ward 1		Ward 2	
	Kappa	%	Kappa	%	Kappa	%
Task	¥	90.47	¥	91.66	¥	100.00
When	0.71 (ns)	94.40	0.98 ($p<0.001$)	99.05	0.80 ($p<0.001$)	86.27
Duration	¥	79.66	¥	81.57	¥	91.30
Body area	0.83 ($p<0.001$)	85.71	0.90 ($p<0.001$)	91.83	0.73 ($p<0.001$)	77.10
Patient's position	0.76 ($p<0.001$)	80.85	0.83 ($p<0.001$)	90.76	0.95 ($p<0.001$)	97.34
Nurse's position	0.72 ($p<0.02$)	80.85	0*		98.46	0.74 ($p<0.06$)	93.96
Type of touch	0.48*	72.68	0.64 (ns)	87.75	0.42*	85.40
Response	0.53 (ns)	66.44	0.25 (ns)	52.45	0.59*	76.11
Verbal communication	0.39 (ns)	55.97	0.55*	73.43	0.40 (ns)	57.93
Length	0.39 (ns)	59.10	0.40 (ns)	69.56	0.26 (ns)	63.90

* Not enough variation in data for accurate kappa calculation.
¥ Categories unsuitable for kappa calculation; % agreements only calculated.
ns not significant.

Table 1 shows both kappa coefficients and percentage agreement for ten schedule components, of which seven were consistently acceptable (using Cichetti's, 1984, criterion):

(i)   The task being performed, or nature of the interaction
(ii) When the touch occurred in the interaction.
(iii) The duration of the interaction.
(iv) The body area touched.
(v)   The patient's position.
(vi) The nurse's position.
(vii) The type of touch.

Three components, in one setting (when, video; touch type, Ward 1; and nurse's position, Ward 2) each had kappa coefficients of >0.60 but their levels of significance did not reach $p <0.05$. This suggests that Cichetti's criterion might need to be reconsidered.

The three other components had low kappa coefficients and percentages:

(viii)   The response to the touch.
 (ix)   The type of verbal communication by the toucher.
  (x)   The estimated length of each touch episode.

These last three components require subjective judgement and are open to different interpretation by observers. They were, however, retained in the schedule, but in addition to (viii) and (ix) we are recording at the end of each nurse–patient interaction a general comment about its content, speed and communication patterns. This information is used to form an overall picture of the communication occurring during the total interaction rather than for each single touch episode. Recording of the length of each touch may improve with more practice.

Type of Touch

Analysis of the type of touch observed has been completed for four long-term care wards. Thirty patients were observed in these wards and a total of 1420 touches were recorded during 318 interactions, of which 1216 (85.63 per cent) touches were instrumental, 181 (12.75 per cent) were expressive and 23 (1.62 per cent) indefinable. These results strongly suggest that most nurse–patient touch in long-term care wards is instrumental in nature.

Methods for Aim 2

Biographical details for all observed patients and nurses are recorded on the demographic data sheet shown in Figure 2. Recorded are those variables which have been shown in earlier research to affect the use and acceptance of touch (Porter, 1983).

An attempt is also being made to assess old people's preferences for using and for receiving touch. During individual interviews with each observed patient and nurse, we show them pairs of monochrome photographs featuring a nurse and a patient. In each pair of photographs the nurse–patient communication is similar except that in one of each pair the nurse is touching the patient (Figure 3). Subjects are asked to indicate which photograph in each pair they prefer and to give reasons for their choice. We hope that this approach will encourage nurses and patients to discuss their feelings about touch without questioning them directly about it.

PATIENT I.D. CODE

SEX M/F

MEDICAL DIAGNOSIS ....

....

REASON FOR ADMISSION ....

....

DATE OF PRESENT ADMISSION ....

ETHNIC GROUP

- ASIAN ☐
- CAUCASIAN ☐
- MIDDLE-EASTERN ☐
- NEGRO ☐
- ORIENTAL ☐

AGE ....

PAST OCCUPATION ....

(Husband's ....)

MARITAL STATUS S/M/W/D/

RELIGION ....

NURSE I.D. CODE ....

SEX M/F

STATUS

- STUDENT ☐
- STAFF NURSE ☐
- SISTER ☐
- AUXILIARY ☐
- RELIEF / BANK ☐
- AGENCY ☐
- OTHER ☐

ETHNIC GROUP

- ASIAN ☐
- CAUCASIAN ☐
- MIDDLE-EASTERN ☐
- NEGRO ☐
- ORIENTAL ☐

AGE

- 18 - 21 ☐
- 22 - 30 ☐
- 31 - 40 ☐
- 41 - 50 ☐
- 50+ ☐

MARITAL STATUS S/M/W/D

Figure 2 The demographic data sheet

Method for Aim 3

Kogan's Old People Scale (Kogan, 1961) is being used to determine the observed nurses' attitudes towards elderly people. Respondents are asked to record the degree to which they agree or disagree with 34 statements (17 are positively phrased and 17 are negatively phrased) for example:

'Most old people are very relaxing to be with.'
'Most old people make one feel ill at ease.'

The nurses' scores from this scale will be related to their use of touch. This will enable us to establish whether nurses' attitudes towards old people affect the frequency with which they touch during nursing care and the type of touch they use.

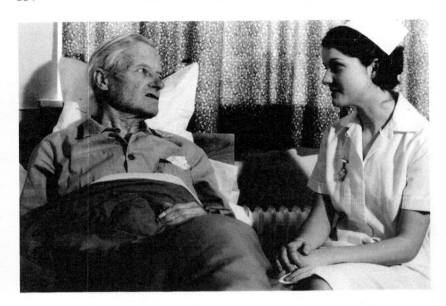

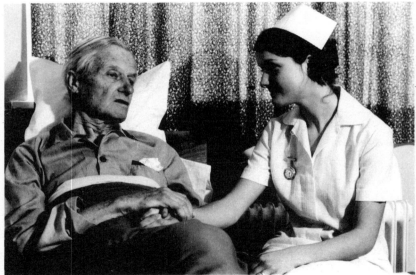

Figure 3   Photographs showing examples of nurse–patient communication.
Reproduced with permission.

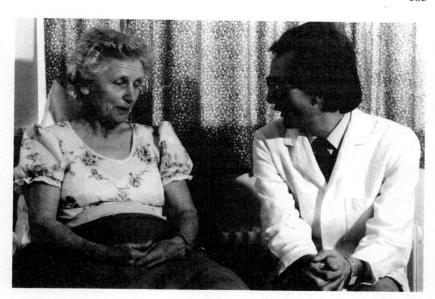

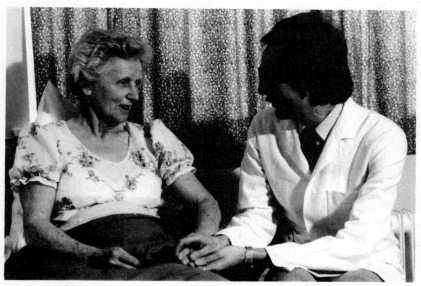

Methods for Aims 4 and 5

Dependency is assessed using the modified version of The Crichton Royal Behavioural Rating Scale (Charlesworth and Wilkin, 1982). This is a ten-item scale designed for use with elderly people. It enables the patient's psychological and physical functional ability to be assessed, as shown in the following examples:

'Feeding   0 Correct unaided at appropriate times
           1 Adequate with minimum of supervision
           2 Inadequate unless continuously supervised
           3 Requires feeding.'

and

'Memory   0 Complete
          1 Occasionally forgetful
          2 Short-term loss
          3 Short and long-term loss.'

This scale is completed by the researcher using information given by the nurse-in-charge.

Patient well-being is assessed with three measures:

(a) The Affect Balance Scale (Bradburn, 1969) which consists of ten items, five of which measure the patient's negative affect (unhappiness) and five positive affect (happiness). For example:

'Today have you felt:
On top of the world?   — Yes/No
Depressed or very unhappy?   — Yes/No.'.

(b) The Wellbeing Scale (Redfern, Porter and Le May 1984) was designed for this study and aims to assess happiness or well-being (Figure 4). This scale was developed with the help of a sample of elderly people, and has not yet been validated.

Both scales are completed by each observed patient, with the interviewer's help if necessary, once on two separate days. The Wellbeing Scale will be validated against the Affect Balance Scale.

(c) Patient engagement/disengagement can also be an indicator of well-being, and an adapted version of a technique used by Felce *et al.* (1980) is being used to assess group and individual patient's engagement levels. Patients are recorded as 'engaged' if they are taking part in some observable activity with another person (e.g.

Please put a tick to indicate how much you feel the way described today

	Not at all	A little	Quite a bit	Extremely
PLEASED				
SATISFIED				
HAPPY				
CONTENT				
CONFIDENT				

Figure 4   The Wellbeing Scale

talking with, or touching), with an object (e.g. reading a book, watching the television, or knitting), or are involved in daily living activities (e.g. washing or dressing), or mobilizing using special aids (e.g. walking frame, rope ladder).

Analysis of the data is in progress. The appropriateness of the outcome measures used to assess dependency and well-being will be established, and any relationship between dependency, well-being and touch will be identified.

This study describes the nature and frequency of touch between nurses and old people in institutional settings for the elderly. It also identifies variables important in touch behaviour, and any relationship between touch and well-being will be determined. The tools used in this research to measure touch and its associated variables may emerge as sufficiently valid for replication by others. If a positive relationship is found between nurses' expressive touch and the well-being of elderly patients, then an increase in the use of appropriate expressive touch should be advocated. Touch is one component of communication skills which should be included explicitly in all nurse training programmes.

Acknowledgement

Andrée Le May is funded through a DHSS Nursing Research Studentship Scheme award. We are grateful to the medical and nursing management of the hospitals who gave us access to do the study, and to the patients and nurses who allowed us to observe them.

References

Aguilera, D. C. (1967). Relationship between physical contact and verbal interaction between nurses and patients. *Journal of Psychiatric Nursing*, Jan/Feb, 13–17.

Barnett, K. (1972a). A theoretical construct of the concepts of touch as they relate to nursing. *Nursing Research*, **21**, 2, 102–110.

Barnett, K. (1972b). A survey of the current utilization of touch by health team personnel with hospitalized patients. *International Journal of Nursing Studies*, **9**, 195–209.

Bowlby, J. (1958). The nature of the child's tie to his mother. *International Journal of Psychoanalysis*, **39**, 350–373.

Bradburn, N. M. (1969). *The Structure of Psychological Wellbeing*. NORC Aldine Publishing Co., Chicago.

Burnside, I. M. (1973). Touching is talking. *American Journal of Nursing*, **73**, 12, 2060–2063.

Burnside, I. M. (1981). *Nursing and the Aged*, 2nd edn. McGraw-Hill Book Co., New York.

Burton, A. and Heller, L. G. (1964). The touching of the body. *The Psychoanalytic Review*, **51**, 1, 122–134.

Charlesworth, A. and Wilkin, D. (1982). *Dependency among Old People in Geriatric Wards, Psychogeriatric Wards and Residential Homes. 1977–1981*, Research Report No. 6, University of Manchester, Psychogeriatric Unit.

Cichetti, D. V. (1984). On a model for assessing the security of infantile attachment: issues of observer reliability and validity. *The Behavioral and Brain Sciences*, **7**, 149–150.

Cohen, J. (1960). A co-efficient of agreement for nominal scales. *Educational and Psychological Measurement*, **20**, 1, 37–48.

Copstead, L. E. (1980). Effect of touch on self appraisal and interaction appraisal for permanently institutionalised older adults. *Journal of Gerontological Nursing*, **6**, 12, 747–752.

De Augustinis, J., Sani, R. S. and Kumler, F. R. (1963). Ward study: the meaning of touch in interpersonal communication, in S. Burd and M. Marshall (Eds), *Some Clinical Approaches to Psychiatric Nursing*. Macmillan, New York.

De Wever, M. K. (1977). Nursing home patients' perception of nurses' affective touching. *Journal of Psychology*, **96**, 163–171.

Dominian, J. (1971). The psychological significance of touch. *Nursing Times*, 22 July, 896–898.

Ernst, P. and Shaw, J. (1980). Touching is not taboo, *Geriatric Nursing (New York)*, **1**, 3, 193–195.

Evers, H. K. (1986). Care of the elderly sick in the United Kingdom, in S. J. Redfern (Ed.), *Nursing Elderly People*. Churchill Livingstone, Edinburgh.
Felce, D., Powell, L., Jenkins, J. and Mansell, J. (1980). Measuring activity of old people in residential care. *Evaluation Review*, **4**, 371–387.
Goodykoontz, L. (1979). Touch: attitudes and practice. *Nursing Forum*, **18**, 10, 4–17.
Henley, N. (1973). Status and sex: some touching observations. *The Bulletin of the Psychonomic Society*, **2**, 41–93.
Hollinger, L. M. (1980). Perception of touch in the elderly. *Journal of Gerontological Nursing*, **6**, 12, 741–746.
Kogan, N. (1961). Attitudes towards old people. The development of a scale and an examination of its correlates. *Journal of Abnormal and Social Psychology*, **62**, 44–54.
Langland, R. M. and Panicucci, C. L. (1982). Effects of touch on communication with elderly confused clients. *Journal of Gerontological Nursing*, **8**, 3, 152–155.
Lorensen, M. (1983). Effects of touch in patients during a crisis situation in hospital, in J. Wilson-Barnett (Ed.), *Nursing Research: 10 Studies in Patient Care*. Wiley, Chichester.
Mehrabian, A. (1972). *Non-Verbal Communication*. Aldine Publishing Co., Chicago.
Montagu, A. (1971). *Touching — The Human Significance of the Skin*. Columbia University Press, New York.
McCorkle, R. (1974). 'Effects of touch on seriously ill patients. *Nursing Research*, **23**, 2, 125–132.
OPCS (1983). Mid year estimates for the United Kingdom. Personal Communication (1984).
Porter, L. (1983). *Development of an Observation Schedule for Recording Nurse-Patient Tactile Communication: an Ergonomic Approach Using Task Analysis*, MSc Thesis, University of London.
Porter, L., Redfern, S., Wilson-Barnett, J. and Le May, A. (1986). The development of an observation schedule for measuring nurse–patient touch, using an ergonomic approach. *International Journal of Nursing Studies*, **23**, 1, 11–20.
Preston, T. (1973). When words fail. *American Journal of Nursing*, **73**, 12, 2064–2066.
Redfern, S., Porter, L. and Le May, A. (1984). The effects of touch on patient's physical and psychological wellbeing: a feasibility study to develop methods. RCN Research Society Annual Conference (25th), London (In Press).
Rubin, R. (1963). Maternal touch. *Nursing Outlook*, **11**, 828–831.
Seaman, L. (1982). Affective nursing touch. *Geriatric Nursing*, **3**, 162–164.
Watson, W. H. (1975). The meanings of touch: geriatric nursing. *Journal of Communication*, **25**, 3, 104–112.
Whitcher, S. J. and Fisher, J. D. (1979). Multidimensional reaction to therapeutic touch in a hospital setting. *Journal of Personality and Social Psychology*, **37**, 1, 87–96.
Wilkin, D. and Jolley, D. J. (1978). Mental and physical impairment in the elderly in hospital and residential care. *Nursing Times*, **74**, 29, 117–120 and 30, 124.

Research in the Nursing Care of Elderly People
Edited by P. Fielding
© 1987 John Wiley & Sons Ltd

CHAPTER 9

Multidisciplinary Education — a Way for the Future?

JENIFER NEWMAN

Introduction

The team approach to care is not new and has been considered for many years as an effective way of dealing with the many problems that may occur in old age. Hills Maguire (1985) states that this is 'popular in theory but difficult to implement in practice'. Evers (1981), in her study of the multidisciplinary team in action in geriatric wards, confirms that 'the notion of team work is poorly defined, and supposed benefits for patients are not always readily apparent'. She also concluded that

> very often, work with patients is co-ordinated not by mutual collaboration amongst a team of equals, but by means of established work routines which are broadly applied to whole categories of patients, and by the operation of the traditional hierarchy of social relations in health care.

'The traditional hierarchy' is described (Peplau, 1971) as a pyramid with nurses positioned at the base and doctors at the very top so that the doctor quite frequently exercises control of treatment although he may have little contact with the patient. This is not real teamwork and it is much criticized. Professor Baroness McFarlane, in her work for the Royal Commission on the National Health Service (1980) confirms this with her conclusions that 'difficulties seen in a multidisciplinary approach are more attributable to interprofessional jealousies than anything more solid'. She pointed out that the areas of conflict in multidisciplinary teams were the same whether they worked in hospital or in the community:

(a) *Leadership* Who is to lead the team? Does it have to be the doctor? Does it have to be the same person all the time?

(b) *Responsibility* There should be a corporate responsibility to the team but each professional has an individual responsibility. There is a legal responsibility. Traditionally, doctors are recognized by the Courts as being legally responsible but this appears to be changing and may need clarification.

(c) *Confidentiality* In a team approach more people have access to information about the patient and this carries some risk with it.

She felt that these difficulties were not insurmountable if properly addressed but so often they are not.

The question of leadership is a major cause of contention. In her research into the different ways that small groups work, Abercrombie (1966) identifies that in a discussion it is not really necessary for a group to have a leader but that if a group has a task to perform it can be accomplished more effectively if there is a leader. She also describes different leadership styles: the one which conforms best to the descriptions of health teams is where all information comes to the leader and he distributes all information. In this case the leader has a very satisfying job but the other members of the group may be discontented. Johnson and Johnson (1982) recognized that usually groups or teams have at least two basic objectives:

1 To carry out and complete a task.
2 To maintain collaborative relationships within the group.

In health care teams the task is the restoration to health or the rehabilitation of the patient and this should be central to the thinking of each member. However, the difficulties of maintaining the 'collaborative relationship' often get in the way of patient care. Traditionally the doctor has been the leader but with the growth of the other health professions, as the result of more highly developed training, it is questionable whether doctors should continue to lead all the time as there will be aspects of care where the doctor is not particularly the most appropriate person to judge the patient's best interests. It has been suggested that the leadership role should be determined by the patient's needs (McFarlane and Batchelor, 1980) but unenlightened adherence to traditional hierarchical roles can prevent this happening especially when there is a belief that if leadership is awarded 'on the basis of ability, education and experience, the doctor in a team would usually (though not always) be the obvious choice', (Salisbury, 1986).

With new education programmes there are many people who are quite able to lead, chair or co-ordinate the team but the doctor may refuse to relinquish the role which he regards as his. This arrogant attitude is not atypical: professional people, especially doctors, who feel they have much to lose if they become a member of a team, may become defensive about their status and behave in a dictatorial fashion. If the doctor continues to hold on to leadership at all times he may achieve satisfaction with his job, ignoring the fact that the remainder of the team are unhappy and dissatisfied. This kind of behaviour is detrimental to a proper approach to whole person care and may serve to reinforce doubts about the existence of a true multidisciplinary team.

A working group at a conference on Medical Education (Earl, 1980) addressed the subject of responsibility in multidisciplinary health care. They concluded for success in this area it was necessary to 'recognize and mutually respect two types of responsibility in the team: the medical responsibility of the doctor and the professional responsibility of the allied worker', which seems to agree with some of what McFarlane and Batchelor (1980) says but does not address the topic of legal responsibility.

Over the past 25 years there have been a few articles written and papers given in an attempt to persuade different disciplines in the health professions to change their methods of training and to run interdisciplinary programmes in health care. The majority appeared in the 1970s (Leninger, 1971; Scott-Wright, 1976; Parkes, 1977; Hutt, 1980). Apparently little change has taken place as Hills Maguire is still making the same pleas in 1985. She states that the 'interdisciplinary approach must begin with the academic and clinical education of health care professionals if we expect to see it functioning in practice' but comments that few educational programmes are interdisciplinary. These papers and books have been written mainly by nurses who, it could be argued, have a vested interest in raising the status of their profession. However, it may be more likely that doctors, with their traditionally privileged status could believe that they had something to lose by participating in courses of this kind. Disputes of this kind have gone on for far too long. Whilst, as students, they are all educated in isolation, a lack of knowledge of the different disciplines will lead to a lack of understanding and respect, interprofessional competition and a stereotyping of roles (Leninger, 1971). Together with Scott-Wright (1976) and Parkes (1977) she stated that everybody should believe in the importance of their contribution to which Scott Wright (1976) added that this would enable them to contribute with confidence to the care of the patient. Only in this way will it be possible to have 'high quality, readily accessible, reasonably comprehensive, co-ordinated, efficient health and welfare services' (Parkes, 1977). These people state, quite rightly, that to achieve this will require changes in education and before there can be a change in education there will have to be a change in attitudes and in behaviour.

There is a great resistance to change and many barriers are erected to avoid it. Too often people say 'It won't work' and refuse to attempt something new. One of the reasons given in the case of multidisciplinary teaching is that the programme would cost too much to run. However, if all health personnel were taught together for parts of their course there would be efficient use of the expertise of highly trained people and a pooling of resources so that the joint education programme would quickly become cost effective.

One of the qualities necessary for running such courses, as Leninger (1971) observed and Yeaworth and Mims (1973) included in their article, is a sense of commitment to the concept. This should be held by all the teachers. These authors suggest that lack of it may account for the failed attempts at this type of teaching. It is impossible to run multidisciplinary courses without considerable investment of time and effort. The tutors and organizers must regard the venture as exciting and promising and efforts should be made to reassure and help those who feel threatened or confused by the changes. Only in this way can they and their students learn to work effectively and interdependently and learn what hinders and what helps group discussion.

The attempts to put theory into practice have also been few. North America and Australia have pursued the idea most assiduously. In Australia, for instance, Bill Pickett wrote in 1976 about the first two years at The Foundation for Multidisciplinary Education in Community Health. This was a co-operative venture by the South Australian Institute of Technology, the University of Adelaide and the South Australian Hospitals Department — all those who were responsible for the education of medical, nursing, physiotherapy, occupational therapy and social work students — and was funded by the Hospitals and Health Services Commission of the Commonwealth and the Hospitals Department of South Australia. In the first instance this was a feasibility study but it became apparent that 'the desirability and urgency of such joint educational activities' had been demonstrated. The emphasis here was on active participation. Certainly nothing is really learnt about the other health professions from sitting together in the same lectures. The students learned, as they usually do in this setting, not only from their teachers but from one another. At this college the unique qualities of the different professions were highlighted as well as the necessary overlap of roles and ensured that everyone realized the importance of their individual contribution.

'The importance of making the patient central to her/his own treatment' is emphasized by Scott-Wright (1976). It is obvious from the papers by Wallgren-Pettersson et al. (1982) in Finland and by Turnbull (1981) writing on a Community Health programme in the United states that the 'pay-off' from participating in an interdisciplinary course is not just for the students but for the patients and for their relatives as well. The course in Community Paediatrics (Wallgren-Pettersson et al., 1982) not only increased the students' awareness of the need for co-operation between the disciplines but made everybody involved aware of the isolation of the parents of a chronically sick child. The whole venture led to more involvement of the parents, better communication and correction of deficiencies in the patients' treatment. As a result the writers felt that this method of learning was important for future health professionals and that a 'greater part of the curriculum should be reserved for interdisciplinary teaching'. This view is reinforced by Croen, Hamerman and Goetzel (1984) from Albert Einstein Hospital in New York who wrote about a programme for medical and nursing students where the care of their elderly patients benefited from improved communication between the disciplines. The writers of this paper realized that common learning experiences are necessary to avoid misunderstandings. During the first two years of their programme it became evident that sometimes the two disciplines did not speak the same language: each had their own jargon and this was a barrier to effective communication.

Rosenaur and Fuller (1973) wrote of the inability of nurses to define or state their role and how this difficulty is a handicap in a team setting. To counteract this, the nursing faculty in their school held a seminar to discuss the nurses' role in primary care to enable future nurses to be more self-confident and able to 'initiate a team relationship' with the medical students. This is an important aspect of nurse training. So often nurses are ill-prepared in the field of communication (Gott, 1983) and this makes it difficult for them to cope with confrontation from others in the health professions and even harder to see themselves as equal members of a team.

In an effort to try to 'explode' some of the myths perpetuated by lack of knowledge of each health care discipline, and to understand how professional rivalry and poor communication can lead to conflict, two psychologists (Brunning and Huffington, 1985) ran a multidisciplinary workshop where each participant took on the role of another discipline and spent the day in that role trying to describe the problems they experienced in the work setting. The results highlighted the difficulties of clearly defining all roles except perhaps the doctor's. This led to uncertainties about people's own role and that of others in the team setting. The writers of the paper felt that if more time were invested on clarifying roles, time spent with the patients would be more productive. In other words the patients would be more firmly established in the centre of everyone's thinking. The authors were disappointed that there were no dramatic changes as a result of this workshop but most change occurs gradually as ways of implementing it became more obvious and less threatening.

Lack of commitment or commitment to a different ideal can seriously hamper the development of interdisciplinary courses. In their paper 'Interprofessional Education in Medical School', Rezler and Gianni (1981) state that previous limited success in the area was due to lack of faculty support and at their medical school, since two-thirds of the male and nearly one-half of the female students were opposed to this type of education they felt that compulsory interprofessional education might be counter-productive. This paper seems to indicate that the authors feel that the purpose of interprofessional education is to show medical students how they can make better use of the other professions: they advocate that attending doctors should 'encourage residents to turn to health professionals, without medical training, for services they either can not, or do not have time to perform'. This perpetuation of the image of health workers other than doctors as the helpers is unacceptable: it does not place the patient as the central figure and reinforces the image of health workers, other that the doctor as 'hand-maidens'. While such attitudes persist there will never be effective teamwork.

Jennifer Gomes in her prize-winning essay (1985) states that all health workers should have some form of common core training: medical, nursing and physiotherapy schools and others too should get together, instead of working in isolation, and plan a common core which would be an integral part of all health students' training. Its most important contribution would be to help to overcome the interprofessional competition which has been observed by so many writers. A move like this would 'make better use of human and natural resources' and would 'allow the health professional to focus all her attention on the patient rather that spend time wastefully on professional "one-upmanship" '.

While people continue to live or work together there will always be conflicts of style, habits and interests. For conflict is an integral part of human existence. When it is avoided, irritations remain unexpressed. This can lead to bad feeling, dissatisfaction and even misery. In order to manage conflict people have to learn 'skills of stating preferences, communicating unambiguously, confronting differences, looking for solutions that make winners of both parties' (Hopson and Scally, 1981). Nowhere do these skills have to be learned more than when people from different backgrounds and with different types of training have to work together.

The professional barriers are getting in the way of successful patient care. The numbers of people over eighty are increasing (OPCS, 1986). Many will ultimately need help. If these people are to receive quality of care and have quality of life their carers must work together harmoniously. Therefore, as a training for professional life, students from different disciplines should have shared learning experiences. This opportunity has been available at the Middlesex Hospital for several years. The multidisciplinary course in Care of the Elderly and its evaluation are now described.

A Multidisciplinary Course in Care of the Elderly and Community Medicine

The original idea for a course of this kind came from the participants at a conference for health students in March 1975. In discussion it was decided that students from different health disciplines would benefit from learning with one another and from one another. This method of learning would help to break down the barriers which exist between the different health professions and which can get in the way of appropriate patient care.

The students began negotiations with the Director of Nurse Education, the Dean of the Medical School and the Consultant Geriatrician. Care of the Elderly involves so many people from different health professions it was considered a suitable area in which to begin this method of training. As a result of these discussions, a course for medical and nursing students to study Care of the Elderly together began in January 1976. A few months later they were joined by physiotherapy students.

The course described began as a multidisciplinary course in Geriatrics (Beynon *et al.*, 1978) but with the formation of a new joint clinical school of medicine (University College and the Middlesex Hospital), the time allocated includes an integral week of Community Medicine. Medical, nursing and physiotherapy students, and occasionally occupational therapy and social work students, learn together for a period of four weeks. The course takes place during the fourth year (second clinical year) of the medical students' training. The nursing students are in the middle of their second year of training and attend either before or after their attachment to a ward for elderly patients. The physiotherapy students are in their third and final year and attend during their placement with elderly patients.

This form of education has been supported since its instigation by the Schools of Medicine, Nursing and Physiotherapy and by the students themselves. The people who teach on the course find the experience challenging. Their commitment has enabled the course to continue to develop over the years to include students and tutors from other disciplines, to embrace new teaching methods and to be open to suggestions for change from everyone involved.

Course Design

The objectives for the course have always been subject to rigorous review and have been changed as the course has developed (Beynon *et al.*, 1978; Hutt, 1980), for a process of reappraisal and development of aims is essential to any new curriculum (Hamilton, 1976). They were reviewed yet again, when the Schools merged and a new curriculum began, to embrace the integration with Community Medicine, and to include some contribution from the Department of General Practice. The objectives are listed in Table 1.

The overall design of the course has been based on these objectives and on the following conditions which are necessary to optimize learning (Warren Piper, 1982):

1   Student knows what is to be learned and wants to learn it.
2   Student knows what she/he has learned.
3   Student practises application.
4   'Errors' are diagnosed quickly, 'treatment' offered.
5   Student is active.
6   Pace is suited to individuals.
7   Student is given a variety of experiences.

Table 1   Aim and objectives

Aim

To enable students from several disciplines to learn together the principles involved in the management of elderly people in hospital and in the community.

Objectives

By the end of the course the students shall
1   be able to demonstrate the principles involved in the management of elderly people in hospital and in the community.
2   be aware that communication with everybody involved (this includes the patient, relatives and/or friends) is essential when rehabilitating and treating elderly people.
3   be aware of the importance of early diagnosis and treatment, and of functional assessment, of the elderly.
4   be able to assess the physical, psychological and social needs of the elderly.
5   be aware that any member of the multidisciplinary team is a professional in his/her own right.
6   be able to outline the role of each discipline.
7   be able to refer to the discipline which will give appropriate treatment to enable the elderly person to achieve the best quality of life.
8   be able to describe the organization and function of a geriatric department.
9   be able to state what resources are available for the elderly.
10   be able to mobilize those resources for acute and continuing care in hospital and in the community.

---

8   Student uses ears, eyes and touch.
9   Information presented in words, drawings, formulae.
10 Ideas are 'complete' and related to student's previous ideas.
11 Student learns to work independently of teacher.

A multidisciplinary course needs to be run by people who are interested in this type of education. Efficient use must be made of the allocated four weeks as a greater number of people are expected to live longer (OPCS, 1986) and many of health students in training will come into contact with old people in their professional life. The students must be encouraged to take a positive attitude towards ageing and old age and must be given every opportunity to see as much as possible of the problems of old age, how they should be managed and what resources are available. Plenty of time must be allowed for informal discussion with one another and with their teachers. The organizer must arrange a sequence of learning which must fit in with the student's needs and the availability of teachers and must try to ensure that the teachers include all the disciplines in their teaching. However, in a multidisciplinary course, the organizer has a wider role. For the students and for new teachers, the course is different. Each may require support and encouragement while they are in a period of adjustment. The organizer must be prepared to help, if necessary, to sort out external difficulties which may be getting in the way of adjustment. Teachers and students may need support too when trying out new teaching methods while the students may need support, because of preconceived ideas, when beginning to work with elderly people.

Course Content

The teachers on the course come from many disciplines and cover a wide variety of topics (Tables 2 and 3).

The first week is an introductory week. Students are introduced to basic concepts in lectures which are complemented by ward rounds, seminars and problem-solving sessions. They are each allocated three or four patients and expected to get to know them and to monitor their treatment and progress. Before the students go to see their patients they are shown lifting techniques as they are frequently quite worried about moving frail elderly patients.

Most of the second week is spent out of the hospital visiting old people in homes, in the community, in continuing care units, a day centre and day hospitals — one for the physically disabled and another

Table 2   Teachers

Doctors
    Consultant geriatricians
    Consultant psychiatrist with a special interest in the elderly
    Senior registrars
    Senior lecturer
    Senior house officers
    General practitioners
Nurses
    Tutor/course organizer
    Ward sisters
    Staff nurses
    Geriatric visitor
    Psychiatric nurse
Social workers: members of the specialist team for the elderly
Physiotherapists
Occupational therapists
Speech therapist
Members of the Department of Anatomy and Biology
Members of the Department of Community Medicine

Table 3   Topics

Introduction to the course
Introduction to geriatric medicine
Introduction to community medicine
Demography
Examination of elderly patients
Life-history taking
Non-specific presentation of illness in old age
Disease patterns in the elderly
Incontinence and incontinence aids
Nursing elderly patients
Stroke illness
Cardiovascular disease
Physiotherapy
Lifting techniques
Occupational therapy
Speech therapy
Social work
Rehabilitation
Continuing care
Care of the elderly in General Practice
Social awareness and attitudes
Family pressures
Ethics
Bereavement
Psychiatric problems of old age
Accidental hypothermia
Drug treatment of the elderly
Falls, funny turns and fractures
The biology of ageing
Survey methods

for elderly people with psychiatric problems. These visits are interspersed with discussion and ward work.

The third week is arranged so that the students can spend their time on the wards talking to and examining their patients, attending the outpatient department and ward rounds and preparing and giving seminars.

The final week is one of consolidation and includes an afternoon spent considering care of the elderly in the community with a general practitioner and a geriatric visitor, and discussion of the problems of carers and of bereavement. All students are required to write an essay which is handed in and marked in the final week. Although titles are suggested e.g. 'Should Geriatrics exist as a separate speciality or should it be integrated with other medical disciplines?' or 'Discuss the importance of health education in the promotion and maintenance of health of the elderly', they may write on any aspect of care of the elderly that they choose provided it takes a broad view.

On the last day the students complete a multiple choice questionnaire and a problem-solving exercise. It is emphasized that these are not examinations but methods of self-assessment. The discussion, which accompanies the marking and follows as soon as they have completed both papers, is a teaching and learning exercise.

The four-week allocation ends with a small party.

Methods of Learning

The students visit the patients in hospital in interdisciplinary pairs. They exchange skills. They help one another learn. As each person's confidence grows most students enjoy the opportunities for sharing learning experiences with their fellow students, their teachers, the ward staff and especially the patients. For all students are encouraged to feel a responsibility to one another, to the teachers and to the patients so that they become involved and can contribute to the care and rehabilitation of their patients. Listening to patients talking about themselves and the events that have shaped their lives (Johnson, 1978) is considered as important as examining them, so that students are encouraged to think about treatment of the whole person instead of diseases in isolation. Seminars are complemented by ward rounds so that what they learn in the classroom is immediately reinforced by seeing appropriate patients on the wards. Problem-solving sessions are arranged with doctors, nurses, occupational therapists and social workers. The occupational therapists also ensure that the students have experiential learning of disability. In all these activities the different disciplines are encouraged to observe how the various professions involved complement one another and how to make use of this facility. Some of the seminars are presented by the students and for these they are expected to work together in multidisciplinary groups and to share the presentation.

In the past couple of years 'The Ageing Game' (Robertson and Brocklehurst, 1981) has been tried out as a means of promoting discussion amongst the students and raising contentious issues. This game also encourages teamwork.

Teaching and learning is in all directions — teachers learn from one another and from the students. The students learn from each other, from their teachers and from their patients. Undoubtedly one of the most popular learning experiences is the multidisciplinary patient presentation (86 per cent of the students score 1 or 2). It is a problem-solving session and forms the core of the course. This type of presentation is fairly simple to arrange and can be used on its own if a multidisciplinary learning experience needs to be tried out. However, it should not be looked upon as a substitute for a longer course.

The format for this session was developed by a consultant geriatrician, a nurse tutor and the course organizer. Guidelines are given to the students to help them to prepare for it (Appendix). There is one presentation in each week of the course and each presentation embodies some of the knowledge, skills and attitudes the tutors would like the students to gain and develop. Sometimes the students are required to take on the role of a member of a different profession. The atmosphere is usually relaxed which encourages the quieter students to participate. The whole presentation is greatly enhanced by a visit to or from the patient.

The students learn listening and communicating and planning techniques. Questions and suggestions offered by them are considered. Quite frequently this can result in a change of treatment or a new strategy. The students feel involved in the patient's care and feel that what they have to say is of use to both the carers and the patient.

Course Evaluation

At the end of each four-week period the students are asked to complete a form to evaluate the course and are asked for their opinions on all their experiences. Their responses to the objectives can be seen in Table 4. From the absence of low scores it can be seen that the students are enthusiastic about the course and sharing learning experiences with different disciplines. Several students think that this type of teaching should be extended to subjects, other than those listed, like oncology, orthopaedics, rheumatology and paediatrics.

Occasionally, a medical student feels 'held back' by the presence of the other disciplines — although the teachers do not change their standards — and this may affect the rating of the medical content of the course.

The use of educational games is rare in the students' training. They are more accustomed to receiving lectures, and their response to this type of teaching method is mixed. However, those who do appreciate The Ageing Game are enthusiastic in their reception. Other newer

Table 4　Evaluation of course by 98 students

1 = To a very great extent 5 = Not at all					

Response to objectives

Are you now:	1	2	3	4	5
Able to demonstrate the principles involved in the management of elderly people in hospital and in the community.	20	56	20	2	0
Aware that communication with everybody involved is essential when rehabilitating and treating elderly people.	73	23	2	0	0
Aware of the importance of early diagnosis and treatment, and of functional assessment, in the elderly.	52	37	8	1	0
Able to assess the physical, psychological and social needs of the elderly.	15	49	28	6	0
Aware that any member of the multidisciplinary team is a professional in his/her own right.	70	18	9	1	0
Able to outline the role of each discipline.	28	50	18	2	0
Able to refer to the discipline which will give appropriate treatment to enable the elderly person to achieve that best quality of life.	33	51	14	0	0
Able to describe the organization and function of a geriatric department.	18	45	29	5	1
Able to state what resources are available for the elderly.	17	51	25	5	0
Able to mobilize those resources for acute and continuing care in hospital and in the community.	1	39	44	11	3

Table 5　Response to multidisciplinary teaching

Do you feel that teaching of medical, nursing and physiotherapy students together is a good idea?	69	18	8	1	2
Do you think that this method can be used satisfactorily in other disciplines? (Some students either ignored or commented only in this section)					
General medicine	17	19	22	19	16
General surgery	13	15	24	22	19
Psychiatry	34	22	23	6	4
Paediatrics	22	24	19	9	7
Will you recommend this course to your colleagues?	34	42	16	4	0

teaching methods like the use of video film, as a means of enhancing a teaching session, are more popular.

The visits are appreciated because they take the students out of the hospital and enable them to have a much clearer idea of the resources which are available. In discussion of the visits the students reveal a large discrepancy between their expectations and the reality.

At the end of the evaluation form students are asked to name particular things that they disliked or liked. Some medical students are outspoken in their criticism of people who single them out and teach to them alone. Indeed the nursing and physiotherapy students can feel very resentful when they have prepared a presentation but their contribution is ignored. Fortunately this does not happen often as the written evaluation serves as a reminder to those who teach. On the whole other dislikes are few and are confined trivialities such as the lack of air conditioning and the type of coffee provided!

Everybody finds the variety — the mixture of seminars, ward rounds, visits to different hospitals and homes and informal discussions — stimulating. They like being involved and praise the 'good teaching from willing teachers'. The emphasis on attitudes and the discussion of contentious issues, raise many ideas which previously have not been considered. In particular, students begin to think about some of the stereotyped views they had before the course about old age and about each other's profession and this usually makes them realize how pervasive and destructive rigid adherence to these views can be.

Discussion

On the whole the students have integrated well and have found the learning experience useful although it can be substantially different from any other they have had before. The course is highly structured. Some students find the structure confining but as this type of learning experience is new, most of them appreciate the feelings of certainty created by it, and there is still plenty of freedom within that structure to question and to discuss and to learn the skills needed for satisfactory communication. They like the fact that the course is well organized and that their teachers stick to the timetable — and so are encouraged to do the same! This is important as 'the heart of the educational process is in the continual broadening and deepening of knowledge in terms of basic ideas' (Bruner, 1982): students have a limited exposure to the materials they are to learn but somehow this exposure must be made to count in their thinking for the rest of their lives. With the change in demographic trends, most of the students when they qualify, will be required to look after increasing numbers of elderly people although they are exposed to care of the elderly for only a few weeks.

Conclusion

The level of success required to improve the care of elderly people and help them retain their autonomy will not be achieved without some investment in training health personnel to acquire skills and expertise in team work. The World Health Organization (1981) recommended that health care workers should have learning experiences together but, as there is no national commitment to this idea, there are still few multidisciplinary health care programmes. Most team training programmes that do exist are run by the National Health Service at senior management level. However, professional life begins long before this stage is reached and team skills, developed at a senior level, are necessary from the beginning. The development of the skills in team-work should be an intrinsic part of the training of health professionals and it is essential that different concepts, aims and attitudes are identified at student level, before stereotyped ideas are fixed.

Attempts to achieve some form of integration are continually frustrated by the rigidity of the institutions in which health care students are educated. This is partly due to the fact that their teachers, those already in the professions, once they are established in their careers are constrained by various work pressures. Although teachers may become aware of the need for shared learning experiences, they find them difficult to set up, let alone establish, as multidisciplinary courses, require considerable investment of time and effort.

These difficulties are surmounted by resistance to change. Nobody likes change, but if there is to be a health education system which is remotely in touch with the health needs of the late twentieth century, fundamental changes will have to take place. The blinkered approach of many health professionals, which is passed on to their students, cannot be allowed to continue. A course of study should enable students to deepen their understanding and widen their views of a subject; it is not just to learn the facts to pass an exam (although the attitude of many teachers and students might lead people to disbelieve this). Teachers and students must be quite sure of the advantages of changing the method of education and training: they should be aware that understanding and knowing one another better and developing mutual trust improves each person's self-confidence and makes the team a satisfactory and supportive vehicle for its members. These conditions can embrace patients and their relatives so that they become members of the team and feel involved in plans for their care.

The health students of today are the professional carers of tomorrow so they must be educated for tomorrow. This must entail making changes today so that all of us, as we grow older, can anticipate an old age where our autonomy and dignity are retained and where we can feel that our best interests are being served by a well-trained, happy, truly professional team.

References

Abercrombie, M. L. J. (1966). Small Groups, in Brian Foss (Ed.) *New Horizons in Psychology*. Harmondsworth: Penguin.
Beynon, G. P. J., Wedgwood, J., Newman, J. and Hutt, A. (1978). Multidisciplinary education on geriatrics: an experimental course at the Middlesex Hospital. *Age & Ageing*, **7** (4), 193–200.
BMA (1986). *All Our Tomorrows*. British Medical Association.
Bruner, J. J. (1982). *The Process of Education*. Harvard University Press.
Brunning, H. and Huffington, C. (1985). Altered Images. *Nurs. Times*, **81** (31), 24–27.
Clarke, R. and Skeet, M. (1981). *Nursing Care of the Elderly*. World Health Organization.
Croen, L. G., Hamerman, D. and Goetzel, R. Z. (1984). Interdisciplinary training for medical and nursing students: learning to collaborate in the care of geriatric patients. *J. Amer. Ger. Soc.*, **32**, Jan., 56–61.
Earl, F. A. (1980). Working Group A: Multidisciplinary health care and education, *Medical Education*, **14**, suppl. p. 68.
Evers, H. K. (1981). Multidisciplinary teams in geriatric wards: myth or reality. *J. Adv. Nurs.*, **6**, 205–214.
Evers, H. K. (1982). Professional practice and patient care: multidisciplinary teamwork in geriatric wards. *Ageing & Society*, **2**, 1, 57–75.
Gomes, J. (1985). Co-operation through core courses. *Community Outlook*, 31–35.
Gott, M. (1983). The preparation of the student for learning in the clinical setting, in Bryn Davies (Ed.), *Research into Nurse Education*. Croom Helm.
Hamilton, J. D. (1976). The McMaster curriculum. *British Medical Journal*, **1**, 1191–1196.
Hills Maguire, G. (1985). The team approach in action, in Gail Hills Maguire (Ed.) *Care of the Elderly: A Health Team Approach*. Little, Brown, Boston/Toronto.
Hopson, B. and Scally, M. (1981). *Lifeskills Teaching*. McGraw-Hill Book Co., UK.
Hutt, A. (1980) Shared learning for shared care. *J. Adv. Nurs.*, **5**, 389–396.
Johnson, D. W. and Johnson, F. P. (1982). Joining Together, 2nd edn. *Group Theory and Group Skills*. Prentice-Hall, Englewood Cliffs, New Jersey.
Johnson, M. (1978). That was your life: a biographical approach to later life,

in Vida Carver and Penny Liddiard (Eds), *An Ageing Population*. Hodder & Stoughton in association with the Open University Press.

Leninger, M. (1971). This I believe: . . . about interdisciplinary health education for the future. *Nurs. Outl.*, **19**, (2), 787–791.

McFarlane, J. and Batchelor, I. (1980). *Multidisciplinary Clinical Teams*. Secretariat of the Royal Commission on the NHS, Kings Fund Centre.

Office of Population Census and Surveys (1986). *Social Trends*, 16. HMSO.

Parkes, M. E. (1977). The importance of seeing the whole picture. *Austral. Nurs. J.*, **11**, June 20–23.

Peplau, H. (1971), Responsibility, authority, evaluation and accountability of nursing in patient care. *Michigan Nurse*, **44**, 5–7.

Pickett, W. (1977). Multidisciplinary education in health science. *Austral. Nurs. J.*, **7**, Dec., 10–11.

Rezler, A. and Gianni, G. (1981). Interprofessional education in medical school. *Med. Educ.*, **15**, 237–241.

Robertson, D. and Brocklehurst, J. C. (1981). The ageing game: a new teaching method in geriatric medicine. *J. Am. Geriatr. Soc.*, **29**, 576–578.

Rosenaur, J. and Fuller, D. (1973). Teaching strategies for interdisciplinary education. *Nurs. Outl.*, **21**, March, 159–162.

Salisbury, C. (1986). Practice teamwork must be effective. *G. P.*, Jan., 15.

Scott-Wright, M. (1976). *The Relevance of Multidisciplinary Education in the Health Care Team: Nurses and Health Care*. King Edward's Hospital Fund, London.

Turnbull, E. (1981). Health care issues as an interdisciplinary course. *Nurs. Outl.*, **29**, 42–45.

Wallgren-Pettersson, C., Donner, M., Holmberg, C. and Wasz-Hockert, O. (1982). Interdisciplinary teaching of community paediatrics. *Med. Educ.*, **16**, 290–295.

World Health Organization (1981). *Nursing Care of The Elderly*. Document No. 6158B, p. 8.

Warren Piper, D. (1982). *Learning Theory and the Concept of Teaching Expertise*. Centre for Staff Development in Higher Education.

Yeaworth, R. and Mims, F. (1973). Interdisciplinary education as an influence system. *Nurs. Outl.*, **21**, Nov. 696–699.

Appendix: Multidisciplinary Patient Presentation and Problem-solving

A student from each discipline is asked to present for discussion the problems of a patient from the Geriatric Unit.

Guidelines for students:

1   It is essential that a history is taken from the patient by each discipline and that the patient is fully examined.
2   Information may be obtained from the patient and/or his relatives, the case notes, the nursing Kardex, doctors, nursing staff, physiotherapists, occupational therapists, social workers and other members of the team.
3   It will be helpful if you begin your presentation with a verbal picture of the person and some information about his social circumstances. This may be done

by a student from any discipline but is usually best from the particular student presenting the patient's social problems.

4   The presentation should last about 20–30 minutes.

5   All students attending are expected to participate in the discussion of possible solutions to the problems of this particular patient.

6   Communication between all the presenters is essential.

7   Points for discussion may include
    (a) Consideration of:
        Daily living needs and quality of life at home and in the ward
    (b) Multipathology
    (c) Effects of treatment/drug therapy
    (d) Motivation/stimulation
    (e) Management:
        How are we coping with this patient?
        Is this adequate?
        How could we improve our care?
        What are the appropriate plans, both short and long-term for this patient's future?

Day of presentation — before your colleagues arrive:

The representative of each discipline should identify the patient's problems from their point of view and list them, in order of priority, on the board. You should be prepared to state how you intend to sort out each problem.

Please bring along the patient's notes and X-rays.

Research in the Nursing Care of Elderly People
Edited by P. Fielding
© 1987 John Wiley & Sons Ltd

CHAPTER 10

Recent Advances in the Understanding of Dementia

ANGELA SYMONS

Introduction

Dementia has been defined as a global deterioration of mental functioning in its cognitive, emotional and conative aspects (Mayer-Gross, Slater and Roth, 1969), conation being the faculty of volition and desire. Short-term memory loss and lack of concentration may be the first signs, although initially remote memory may be well preserved. Mental alertness wanes and periods of confusion and disorientation ensue. As the disorder progresses, signs become more prominent leading eventually to a profound dysfunction with loss of association for surroundings, total dependence on others for mental and physical needs and shortened life expectancy.

In 1978, dementia was given the label of the 'quiet epidemic' (Editorial, 1978). Approximately 5–10 per cent of persons over the age of 65 (Kay, Beamish and Roth, 1964) and 22 per cent of persons over 80 years (Kay et al., 1970) are suffering from some form of dementia. At present, the disorder has a prognosis of continual degeneration of mental and physical function with no effective treatment. The results are devastating not only for the sufferer but also for the family. The Health and Social Services are already overburdened, with scarce resources for the management of dementia, but the problem will continue to increase due to demographic changes in developed countries. In Britain, over the last 50 years the elderly population has grown substantially faster than the younger population both on account of the fall in birth-rate after the early 1920s and with general improvement of health and social conditions, leading to an increase in the proportion surviving to old age (Wroe, 1978). The population will continue to become older until a new equilibrium is achieved when those people born in the last decades of reduced infant mortality reach old age.

The two main types of dementia are senile dementia of the Alzheimer type (SDAT), so called as its pathology is indistinguishable from true Alzheimer's disease (first used to describe dementia of the pre-senium), and multi-infarct dementia (MID). SDAT is characterized by an insidious onset with continuous downhill progression. The neuropathology macroscopically shows shrinkage of gyri and widening of sulci with cerebral atrophy. Microscopically, typical neurofibrillary tangles and senile plaques can be identified with disappearance of many neurones. MID often has an abrupt onset with stepwise deterioration following repeated cerebrovascular episodes. The neuropathological picture shows degeneration and softening of brain substance with small, unevenly distributed focal infarcts.

The two common forms of dementia have different aetiologies and different associated problems but share a final common pathway of profound mental impairment leading to death. The two disorders are often seen together (mixed dementia), probably not as an association but due to chance since both disorders are fairly common in the elderly.

At present, the causes of senile dementia are poorly understood thus prevention and 'cure' are not possible. Treatment is geared to relief of symptoms as they arise, with support for patients and relatives in the community, and when necessary institutional admission for short reliefs or long-term care.

In recent years, realization of the far-reaching consequences of dementia has prompted a wealth of research, which can broadly be divided into two areas:

1   Elucidation of the primary cause(s) of dementia so that an effective therapy can be sought and preventative measures taken.
2   Understanding of the most effective and efficient methods of management, symptomatic relief and remedial therapies.

Prior to looking at these two areas in more detail, a very important consideration in relation to research into dementia is that of ethics.

Ethics and the Demented Patient

There are certain special ethical considerations in the research of dementia, particularly relating to consent. As with all research on human subjects, prior informed consent must be obtained. Informed consent means that not only has the subject had a thorough explanation of the protocol, but also that he understands his involvement, the risks and benefits and is prepared to participate. Unfortunately, among the cardinal features that are of clinical interest in dementia are loss of insight, intellect and judgement, which are the very faculties necessary for informed consent (Mahendra, 1984).

The 1964 Declaration of Helsinki, revised in 1975, gives guidelines concerning consent in the case of legal incompetence, and advises that permission from a responsible relative, preferably in writing, should replace that of the subject. However, an important point to remember is that the demented subject may or may not be able to consent, but he can refuse and any reticence or unco-operativeness should be regarded as such. Another important point is that all patients 'belong' to their doctors. In the community the general practitioner's consent should be sought, and in hospital this should be obtained from the relevant consultant. The foreseeable risks to a subject from research may appear negligible but the physician in charge may have additional information. 'Risk' and 'harm' in a research context are usually presumed to be caused by physical agents such as surgical or invasive procedures, or pharmacological effects. However, psychological damage to subjects or relatives in dementia research is an important consideration. A recent example from the Southampton study highlights this. A female subject was referred by a psychogeriatric consultant to the study and was visited at home, where she lived with her husband who was also dementing. Both consented to her taking part in the research. The social situation was not fully understood and when the general practitioner was informed, he did not consent to her inclusion into the study. This dementing couple had apparently only recently become known to the primary health care team and many workers had suddenly become involved, i.e. a social worker, the community psychiatric nurse and meals-on-wheels. The GP felt that one more stranger calling at the house may tip the already precarious balance causing further confusion and disorientation. This subject was therefore withdrawn from the study.

Prior to any research on human subjects, a detailed protocol including all information to be given to subjects, procedures, risks and benefits must be submitted to an ethical body for approval. Approval tends to be given according to the presumed risk : benefit ratio. However, it is still the responsibility of the researcher to ensure that subjects, guardians and physicians have the opportunity to refuse consent or withdraw during any part of the study. With longitudinal studies, which are becoming more common in dementia research, it is important to reaffirm verbally at each meeting that the original consent still stands.

In the USA, in 1981 the National Institute on Aging suggested guidelines addressing ethical and legal issues in dementia (Melnick *et al.*, 1984). They discuss many issues, amongst which they advise that wherever possible, subjects who are at an early stage in the disease process should be used, since they still hold a capacity for judgement and choice. They also suggest useful ways of improving consent forms and procedures for the demented patient.

Research into the Causes of Dementia

Epidemiology

Epidemiological studies have yielded some important information on the dementias. As with all studies on dementia, difficulties arise out of inadequacies of information collection because of the very nature of the disorder and reliance must be placed on relatives and carers being good historians. Epidemiological studies tend to highlight areas of possible interest which can be followed more specifically with retrospective and prospective studies.

Prevalence

The importance of prevalence statistics lies with the future planning of health service resources. Accurate determinations can only be made by community screening of a large sample over a wide geographical area since it has been shown that many of these sufferers do not come to the attention of the primary health care team.

The most comprehensive and most frequently quoted studies are those from Newcastle. Kay and his colleagues investigated the prevalence of all forms of mental illness in the aged and found that of organic brain syndromes to be 10 per cent in those over the age of 65 years (Kay, Beamish and Roth, 1964). Breakdown of this figure showed senile brain syndrome (SDAT) to account for 4.2 per cent, arteriosclerotic brain syndrome (MID) accounting for 3.9 per cent and brain syndromes due to other causes in 1.9 per cent of this population. Their follow-up study (Kay *et al.*, 1970) gave a lower prevalence rate of 6.2 per cent for chronic brain syndromes in the over-65 age bracket, reflecting more stringent inclusion criteria. However, they also showed that this rate accelerated to 22 per cent in those aged 80 years and above. Females were found to have an apparently higher prevalence rate than males, SDAT being more common in females but MID being more prevalent in males.

Genetic Studies

In some dementias (Pick's disease and Huntington's chorea) there is evidence of a monogenic inheritance. In SDAT, however, the case is not clear-cut. There does appear to be a weak genetic link. A recent review of genetics, ageing and dementia (Wright and Whalley, 1984) shows that most studies agree on a multifactorial mode of inheritance. However, one study (Larsson, Sjogren and Jacobson, 1963) suggested a single dominant gene with reduced penetrance. Penetrance may be reduced due to the late age of onset (i.e. many relatives die before the disorder shows), and undoubtedly many affected relatives remain undetected in the community. The small increase in risk to relatives as compared with the general population is more easily reconciled with a multifactorial hypothesis.

In MID there have been few satisfactory genetic studies, but it appears that disorders such as hypertension and degenerative vascular disease, which are themselves under some degree of genetic control (Berg, 1983), are thought to be associated with the development of MID. A recent study (Jarvik and Matsuyama, 1983) showed that parental stroke can be a risk factor for MID, which they postulate to be under genetic influence. However, they do stress the importance of not underestimating nutritional and other exogenous influences.

Other Risk Factors

Other epidemiological studies have shown certain risk factors associated with dementia. Heyman *et al.* (1984) have demonstrated an excess of thyroid disease among women with SDAT compared with matched controls, but suggest perhaps an associated autoimmune disorder rather than an effect of altered thyroid activity *per se* on cognitive function. The same study also found an increased frequency of prior serious head trauma (15 per cent compared with 3.8 per cent in control subjects). The trauma occurred 30–40 years before the onset of symptoms and they proposed an altered blood–brain–barrier, thus sensitizing the immune system to specific brain antigens. However, the long delay between events makes this unlikely.

There is little evidence to link dementia with prior viral infections (except in Creutzfeldt–Jacob syndrome), environmental toxins, medications, eating habits or smoking. The Office of Health Economics (Wells, 1979) has reported

> an important negative epidemiological finding is that no evidence has emerged implicating environmental influences such as isolation and poor social conditions. These factors are found in association with senile dementia but appear to be a consequence of the condition rather than having an aetiological bearing on it.

One question which has not yet been resolved is the relationship between aluminium toxicity and dementia. Aluminium has certainly been implicated in dialysis dementia — an irreversible state following dialysis where there is a high concentration of aluminium in the dialysate. No plaques and tanlges are seen in this condition. However, animal experiments have shown that aluminium induces the formation of argyrophylic tangles resembling the tangles of Alzheimer's disease. The possible association of aluminium with dementia produced excitement a few years ago, when aluminium levels were found to be raised in autopsy and biopsy specimens from cases of SDAT (Crapper, Krishnan and Quittkat, 1976). However, there was found to be considerable overlap between diseased and normal brains. Aluminium increases the permeability of the blood–brain–barrier (BBB) to small peptides which are behaviourally active in rat brains (Banks and Kastin, 1983). The authors suggest a neurochemical hypothesis involving memory. Terry (1985) suggested that the aluminium excess in some tissue specimens is an epiphenomenon rather than a causal one since concentrations in brain tissue do correlate with regional concentrations in drinking water. As yet there are no published data on prevalence of dementia in different regions correlated with aluminium content of water.

Silicon concentrations in cerebrospinal fluid have been correlated with severity of functional impairment in patients with late onset SDAT (Hershey, Hershey and Varnes, 1984). However, one explanation they offer is that as silicon is a normal constituent of brain tissue, the raised levels may be a measure of silicon release following neuronal death.

This avenue of research has been revived recently due to availability of more powerful laboratory techniques. Candy et al. (1986) using high-resolution solid-state nuclear magnetic resonance techniques have shown aluminium and silicon to be present as aluminosilicates at the centre of senile plaque cores. The authors suggest that this could be involved in the initiation or early stages of senile plaque formation.

Treatable Causes of Dementia

Much research has shown that the dementia syndrome can occur through causes which are potentially treatable. A recent study (Smith and Kiloh, 1981) showed that of 200 consecutive admissions with a provisional diagnosis of dementia, 3.8 per cent of those aged over 65 had a potentially reversible cause. This highlights the importance of thorough clinical evaluation and good history-taking. The more common treatable causes are outlined below:

— Depression is known to mimic dementia or confound already existing symptoms, commonly termed depressive pseudodementia. Anti-depressant therapy can markedly increase performance in these patients. Obviously any affective component should be taken into consideration when analysing psychometric data in such patients. Other psychiatric disorders, such as paranoid and schizophrenic conditions, will also mask a true picture of dementia.
— Metabolic disorders, the most common being those of thyroid function, can impair cognition. However, in some cases it is unclear whether treatment reverses cognitive dysfunction or merely arrests it.
— Deficiency states, e.g. Vitamin B_{12} deficiency have been associated with mental impairment (Strachan and Henderson, 1965).
— Infectious diseases may predispose to reversible or irreversible dementia. Neurosyphilis is still an important consideration.
— Normal pressure hydrocephalus due to defective absorption of the cerebrospinal fluid in the arachnoid villi and enlarged ventricles, causes a characteristic dementia syndrome with urinary incontinence as an early sign. Treatment where feasible is by neurosurgical insertion of a CSF shunt.

A comprehensive review of treatable causes has been documented in a recent publication (Small and Jarvik, 1982).

Neurophysiological Research

SDAT

Recent research into the cause of SDAT has centred on a deficit of the central cholinergic system which has been implicated in memory. In

1976, Davis and Maloney showed a reduction in choline acetyl-transferase (CAT) in post-mortem cerebral cortex. CAT is a biosynthetic enzyme for acetylcholine and is a useful post-mortem marker of the integrity of cholinergic neurones. The same workers found a reduction in a similar enzyme, acetylcholinesterase (ACE), in those areas of the cerebral cortex with the greatest density of neurofibrillary tangles. Perry et al. (1978) reinforced the cholinergic hypothesis by finding a correlation between reduction of CAT and ACE activities and mean senile plaque count. Reduction of CAT activity also correlated with the extent of intellectual impairment as measured by a memory information test. Adolfsson et al. (1979) found lower concentrations of certain catecholamines in some areas of the brain again suggesting a defect of neurotransmission. This has led to attempts to intervene pharmacologically, by enhancing transmittor release from remaining neurones, or using direct agonists. However, studies using cholinergic precursors such as choline and lecithin (analogous with levodopa in Parkinson's disease) have so far been disappointing (Cohen and Wurtman, 1976, Hirsch and Wurtman, 1978, Brinkman and Gershon, 1983).

MID

It was in 1974 that Hachinski first coined the phrase 'multi-infarct dementia' to segregate deterioration due to vascular lesions as a separate disease entity from SDAT. Before that time it was generally named arteriosclerotic dementia, implying causation, but it was found that there were no differences in atherosclerosis of extracranial or cerebral arteries between demented and non-demented subjects of comparable age.

In recent years many theories have been put forward as to the cause of multiple infarcts. Atherosclerosis is now not thought to be a primary cause. Hypertension is generally accepted to be a predisposing factor, but paradoxically, over-zealous lowering of the blood pressure does not allow time for the cerebral autoregulation curve to adapt. Consequently, cerebral blood flow is reduced.

In a retrospective study of cardiovascular disease and type of dementia (Ratcliffe and Wilcock, 1985), myocardial infarction, valvular disease, heart size and atheroma of the Circle of Willis showed no significant differences between the different diagnostic categories of dementia. However, a strong association was found between atrial fibrillation (AF) and cerebral infarction even though no patients had intracardiac thrombosis — a prime suspect for formation of emboli. The authors suggest that thrombi may be small or transient, or that AF is simply a marker for some other process predisposing to MID.

Cerebral Blood Flow

It is now well established that cerebral blood flow (CBF) in dementia is lower than in normal controls. One study (Hachinski *et al.*, 1975) suggested that MID is associated with a lower overall CBF than is SDAT. There is still much debate as to why this occurs. Some suggest that it is a response by cerebral autoregulatory mechanisms to reduced oxygen demand by already damaged, metabolically underactive brain tissue. Others have attributed it to reduced flow properties of blood, implying that the resultant regional hypoxia is a cause of neuronal death and dementia. There are good arguments for both sides. One study showed parallel changes in regional CBF with regional cerebral metabolic rate for oxygen in a group of normal subjects and one subject with SDAT while performing hand grip exercises (Raichle *et al.*, 1976). They concluded that regional metabolic rate was the determinant of regional CBF, but their use of a single dement and no MID patients makes the conclusion spurious. Thomas *et al.* (1977) showed that following venesection of patients with high haematocrit, CBF was increased by 50 per cent whereas the oxygen carrying capacity of the blood was only increased by 15 per cent, showing that the resultant decrease in the viscosity of the blood was the predominating factor governing CBF.

Following CBF observations in dementia, treatment of MID has mainly centred on trying to increase CBF by two broad methods; either by increasing the flow properties of the blood or by vasodilator drugs. This latter method has not been successful and may actually decrease the blood supply to ischaemic areas of the brain by dilating healthy vessels more than diseased vessels.

Management in Relation to Research

Current management methods advocate keeping the demented patient in the community for as long as possible where there is a carer, i.e. relative or friend. This has partly stemmed from economic factors and bed availability, but also from research on morbidity and mortality associated with relocation. However, there then becomes a need for community support. Relatives are usually prepared to look after their demented dependant providing they have a supportive back-up system.

Many studies have looked at the impact of care-giving on care-givers — their perceptions and problems. Sanford (1975) analysed the reasons behind 50 geriatric admissions to hospital because of a break-down in coping ability at home. The supporters were asked to assess the causes of inability to cope, and identify those factors which, if alleviated, would restore a tolerable situation at home. The problems fell into three groups; dependants' behaviour patterns; supporters' own limitations; environmental and social conditions. Among the depend-ants' behavioural changes, many potential problem areas were iden-tified but some of these were well tolerated. Incontinence of urine occurred frequently but 81 per cent of those who had to deal with this could tolerate it. Faecal incontinence on the other hand, occurred less frequently but was poorly tolerated. The most common 'last straw' for supporters was night disturbance through dependants' wandering, noisy behaviour or nocturnal micturition. Supporters' limitations included physical and mental problems. Anxiety, depression and embarrassment were noted, as were inability to lift, or aid with activities of daily living (ADL) through lack of strength or supporters' own disability. Environmental and social factors included financial disadvantage, inability to leave the dependant, restriction of social life and holidays. Most of these problems can be alleviated with careful thought; an incontinence laundry service for faecal incontinence; reinstitution of regular sleeping habits by daytime stimulation, night sedation, fluid restriction before bedtime, etc.; use of day-care or a granny-sitting service to allow the carer some time alone; aids for the disabled such as commode and bath hoist. Having identified the specific areas where problems arise, it is easy to see that perhaps a checklist of these items could be completed by the carer, and an individual care plan tailored for each patient and carer.

Another recent report (Gilleard, 1985) looked specifically at the effect of day-care for the patient on alleviation of supporters' stress and strain. He highlighted factors associated with stress levels using questionnaires and interviews with supporters and found associations between high stress levels and behavioural disturbances, supporters' poor health, a poor pre-morbid relationship, incontinence, lack of hygiene and poor housing. Not associated with level of reported strain were patients' physical disability, amount of help received, amount of time spent with dependant, length of illness or age of the patient. Some of these factors are inconsistent with the results of Sanford (1975) but the population and assessment methods are not directly comparable. Gilleard's findings raised questions over whether day-care would have an impact, since carers did not view lack of help received and amount of time spent with the patient as particularly stressful. However, the supporters were interviewed 3–4 months after initiation of day-care in the light of eventual outcome. Relatives whose dependants were still attending day-care showed reduced emotional distress, though not as great a reduction as those whose dependants were taken into long-term care. There was no change in those who ceased to attend.

Psychosocial Approaches to Management

There is little hope that, without specific treatment aimed at the primary cause, the progressive downhill path in dementia can be modified. However one psychological treatment approach has recently received considerable attention. Reality orientation (RO) has been developed specifically for confused elderly people. The underlying principle is that the patient is constantly re-orientated with respect to time, place, person and events in the surroundings. It is stressed that confused and rambling talk is not reinforced, but that either the therapist tactfully disagrees, changes the subject or acknowledges the feelings but ignores the content. Promotion of communication is achieved by clear speech, encouragement of responses, use of past experiences as a bridge to the present, use of eye contact and touch to keep attention, encouragement of humour, and by providing a commentary on surrounding events.

Various methods have been adopted to achieve this. Some centres use an intensive approach with small groups for 30 minutes or so each day with an occupational therapist, while others carry this on throughout the day via nursing and remedial staff.

Many studies have investigated the effectiveness of RO and have been reviewed recently (Wood and Holden, 1982). In summary, most controlled trials have found improvements in cognition and/or behaviour following periods of RO. A sessional approach with 24-hour supporting RO is associated with a more positive behavioural improvement. The cessation of RO appears to be associated with regression to the former state, but the time for this to occur varies between studies. Wood and Holden suggest that RO should be envisaged as a permanent part of the environment and not as a short-term treatment. The training of primary carers to institute a RO programme at home may prove to be of some clinical value. However, the repetition involved in constant orientation of a forgetful person may be too stressful and demanding on the carer.

Psychometric Evaluation of the Demented Patient

For clinical purposes, a psychometric test battery is not necessary, and evaluation is often made by use of a short mental status questionnaire. Behavioural and functional assessments are far more pertinent to management than, for instance, is a complex sorting task. However, research often necessitates a detailed evaluation of mental function, so that comparisons can be made pre- and post-treatment, or to correlate against other variables.

There is a vast number of psychometric tests available for measurement of different aspects of dementia. Cognition, memory — both primary and secondary — attention span, behaviour, psychomotor function and activities of daily living all have numerous assessment methods. The more commonly used methods are those of observation, questionnaires for patient and/or carer, memory tests, psychometric tests, i.e. object sorting and rating scales.

Many of these tools are not specifically designed for use with geriatric patients, so their validity in this field is questionable. A recent review of rating scales for geriatric patients (Hamilton, 1982) provides a useful starting point for any researcher interested in this aspect of dementia. When choosing the type of test, it is important to remember that a combination of tests will yield far more information than one general dementia rating scale. There is also enormous variation in ability between demented patients, so the test battery must be easy enough for the severely demented to obtain a score, but not so easy that discrimination is lost at the milder range of dementia. Many problems encountered with psychometric testing are outlined by Piper (1979).

Longitudinal Study

Dementia is not a static disorder but a progressive one, and the associated problems constantly change with that progression. For this reason, many workers have realized that the most useful data on dementia are gained from longitudinal study and follow-up. Sussman (1964) regarded longitudinal design as the most sensitive way to examine an hypothesis about change.

In Southampton, we have undertaken a multidisciplinary longitudinal study to gain further understanding on the natural course of the disorder and to isolate certain factors which may have a bearing on the disease process. To maximize information gained during the progression, our first criterion was to recruit those suffering from dementia in the early stages. Only patients who were newly referred to the psychogeriatric and geriatric services were referred to the study by the specialist consultant, and therefore, most of the subjects were still living in the community.

Each subject was interviewed at the place of residence and consent was obtained from the subject, the primary carer and the GP. General and medical information was obtained from the hospital case notes with the consultant's permission and any additional information was sought from the carer (if there was one) at the time of interview. Interviews were repeated every three months, the time interval being chosen for three reasons. Firstly, the disorder usually progresses slowly so more frequent testing was unlikely to yield further information in the majority of cases. Secondly, more frequent assessment could have reduced the likelihood of compliance and participation over a long period of time — three years in our study. Lastly, having determined subject numbers and duration of each interview, the time interval using only one rater was calculated. The frequency of measurement in relation to subject numbers and study duration has been examined by Schlesselman (1973b).

At each three-monthly visit, recent events and changes in health, circumstance or treatment were ascertained from the carer, and a psychometric test battery was used to assess mental state, the contents of which were decided by using the following criteria:

1   The battery needed to be short and not too tiring. Attention span is often limited in dementia and subjects may have withdrawn or performed poorly if faced with a long barrage of tests on a regular basis.
2   It needed to have high test–retest reliability.
3   Transportability into subjects' homes was a necessity.
4   The tests had to be sensitive enough to detect change, but not so sensitive that they became too complex so that what we gained in fine discrimination was lost due to fatigue and incomprehension.
5   The tests had to be easy enough for the severely demented to obtain a score but not so easy that discrimination was lost at the milder range of dementia.
6   We aimed to compose a battery that was independent of previous

education and intelligence, although for longitudinal study, subjects do serve as their own controls to an extent.

A battery that fulfilled the criteria and gave a wide range of information included the Clifton Assessment Procedures for the Elderly — survey version (Pattie, 1981); memory tests of immediate and delayed free recall using word lists and digit span; psychomotor speed tasks of shape sorting, letter deletion and choice reaction time. This test battery was validated on a stable, long-stay sample in a local hospital as part of a study on post-operative confusion in the elderly (Burrows, Briggs and Elkington, 1985). In this sample there were no significant differences between any of the tests on five consecutive days, showing that not only are these tests reliable indicators of function but also that there is no practice or learning effect. In the longitudinal study a behavioural assessment was also made using the Sandoz Clinical Assessment for Geriatrics (SCAG) which also gives a measure of any affective component to the disorder which will have an effect on test performance.

During the two-year recruitment period, 118 patients were referred to the study. Of these, 11 were not included either because of refusal, or the dementia was too advanced for any initial scores to be obtained, or there was a severe communication difficulty. Of the 107 study subjects, 69 were female and 38 were male. The mean age was 79 years (±6.3 years). Nearly 18 per cent were living at home alone, 28 per cent living with a spouse and 11 per cent with off-spring. A quarter of the subjects were already in care, either warden-assisted, 'part III' or hospital. Twelve per cent were referred to the study when they became in-patients for a medical reason, suggesting that although dementing, they were not yet known to the specialist services.

On admission to the study, the Clifton Assessment Procedures for the Elderly (CAPE) scores showed a wide variation. The overall score has a possible range of +12 (no functional impairment) to −12 (severely demented). The mean sample score was 2.8 (±4.7), showing that some subjects were already severely affected. This gives cause for concern since these patients were all new referrals to the specialist services, and are not coming to light until they are a long way down the road of dementia. There are probably two reasons for late referral; undoubtedly a large proportion remain undetected in the community either because they live alone and the deficit remains undetected, or they are living with relatives who do not see this as a 'medical' problem and are prepared to assume a caring role to shield the dement; secondly, it is known that some GPs do not like to refer, retaining sole responsibility for management, even though the psychogeriatric service promotes early referral for the most effective management strategies.

It is hoped that longitudinal results will yield more information about the dementing process and data are still being collected. One result that is emerging is that the rate of decline varies considerably. Many studies have documented the reduced life expectancy and time course of dementia (Kay, Beamish and Roth, 1962; Kay *et al.*, 1970; Gilmore, 1975). However, this is usually based on information gained post-diagnosis. Many of the study subjects had been progressing for up to ten years before relatives sought help. Others had a history of only a few weeks but progressed rapidly to death. In most cases it is impossible to determine the exact time when the dementing process began.

Problems of Longitudinal Study

Depletion of Study Numbers

With any study over time, depletion of study numbers is an important consideration. In studies on dementia the age factor and increased mortality will significantly decrease study numbers over time. Refusal to continue participating will also be encountered. However, my personal view based on our study is that the subjects tend to enjoy the visits since they often have little social contact and the stimulation provides a deviation from the everyday routine. Carers also find it a welcome break from routine and are usually pleased that someone is showing interest in an area which is not thought to be a glamorous side of health care. Of 107 subjects recruited to the study, only three have withdrawn consent.

Relocation of the subject from home to hospital or other accommodation may or may not deplete numbers depending on the mobility of the researcher. We recruited from a geographical area defined by the city boundaries and were allowed access to all forms of residence. Some subjects were relocated many times during the study but unless they moved out of the city, follow-up continued.

Statistical Analysis

Statistical analysis of longitudinal data is far more complex than that of cross-sectional data. The researcher should have a clear idea of the statistical methods that he/she is going to employ prior to deciding study numbers. Longitudinal data can be viewed as a change with respect to time. The mental status of each subject at recruitment will be different and the rate of change will also vary, some deteriorating quickly while others may take many years. Schlesselman (1973a) suggests that while change with respect to time may be viewed as a straight line for planning purposes, the analysis should not be so restricted and curve-fitting to each individual's data should be employed.

Observation

Ideally, all subjects should be tested by the same rater at each visit. This may be circumvented by using a pilot study to show the inter-rater reliability. However, difficulties do arise when information is sought from the carer, for the following reasons:

1   The carer may want to protect the dependant and conceal his weaknesses for fear that he will be taken into care.
2   The carer paints an exaggerated picture in the hope that the dependant is taken into care.
3   The subject lives in an institution where the rater may see a different carer at each visit.
4   Relocation means that the carer changes. For example, a subject in warden assisted accommodation may be seen as functionally poor whereas the same subject viewed by the staff of a home for the elderly mentally infirm may be considered to have a relatively good performance.

Cognitive assessments often do not rely on the carer's information so the above variables are of no consequence. However, performance will depend on other factors such as comfort. Concentration and co-operation can be maximized by ensuring that the tests are performed in a quiet, private setting, avoiding meal times and ensuring that the bladder has been voided recently! The subject's usual communication aids such as clean glasses, a hearing aid and dentures should always be used.

Dementia is becoming an increasing problem and research into all aspects of the disorder is still needed. Hopefully the end point will be prevention or effective treatment of the majority of dementias, but until such time the most efficient strategies can only be sought if there is a comprehensive base of good quality research.

Acknowledgement

I would like to thank Dr R. S. Briggs for his invaluable assistance throughout the study period, and also in providing help and guidance in the preparation of this chapter.

References

Adolfsson, R., Gottfries, C. G., Roos, B. E. and Winblad, B. (1979). Changes in brain catecholamines in patients with dementia of the Alzheimer type. *Brit. J. Psychiat.*, **135**, 216–223.

Banks, W. A. and Kastin, A. J. (1983). Aluminium increases permeability of the blood–brain barrier to labelled DSIP and B-endorphin: possible implications for senile and dialysis dementia. *Lancet*, **2**, 1227–1229.

Berg, K. (1983). The genetics of coronary artery disease. *Prog. Med. Genetics*, **5**, 35–90.

Brinkman, S. D. and Gershon, S. (1983). Measurement of cholinergic drug effects on memory in Alzheimer's disease. *Neurobiol. Ageing*, **4**, 139–145.

Burrows, J., Briggs, R. S. and Elkington, A. R. (1985). Cataract extraction and confusion in elderly patients. *J. Clin. Exp. Gerontol.*, **7**, 51–70.

Candy, J. M., Klinowski, J, Perry, R. H., Perry, E. K., Fairburn, A., Oakley, A. E., Carpenter, T. A., Atack, J. R., Blessed, G. and Edwardson, J. A. (1986). Aluminosilicates and senile plaque formation in Alzheimer's disease. *Lancet*, **1**, 354–357.

Cohen, E. L. and Wurtman, R. J. (1976). Brain acetylcholine: control by dietary choline. *Science*, **191**, 561–562.

Crapper, D. R., Krishnan, S. S. and Quittkat, S. (1976). Aluminium, neurofibrillary degeneration and Alzheimer's disease. *Brain*, **99**, 67–80.

Davies, P. and Maloney, A. J. F. (1976). Selective loss of central cholinergic neurones in Alzheimer's disease. *Lancet*, **2**, 1403.

Editorial (1978). Dementia — the quiet epidemic. *Brit. Med. J.*, **1**, 1–2.

Gilleard, C. J. (1985). The impact of psychogeriatric day care on the patient's supporting relatives. *Health Bull (Edinb).*, **43**(4), 199–205.

Gilmore, A. J. J. (1975). Some characteristics of non-surviving subjects in a three-year longitudinal study of elderly people living at home. *Geront. Clin.*, **17**, 72–79.

Hachinski, V. C., Lassen, N. A. and Marshall, J. (1974). Multi-infarct dementia — a cause of mental deterioration in the elderly, *Lancet*, **2**, 207–209.

Hachinski, V. C., Hiff, L. D., Zilkha, E., DuBoulay, G. H., McAllister, V. L., Marshall, J., Ross-Russell, R. W. and Symon, L. (1975). Cerebral blood flow in dementia. *Arch. Neurol.*, **32**, 632–637.

Hamilton, M. (1982). Use of rating scales in geriatric patients. *Gerontology*, **28**, Suppl. 2, 42–48.

Hershey, L. A., Hershey, C. O. and Varnes, A. W. (1984). CSF silicon in dementia — a prospective study. *Neurology*, **34**, 1197–1201.

Heyman, A., Wilkinson, W. E., Stafford, J. A., Helms, M. J., Sigmon, A. H.

and Weinberg, T. (1984). Alzheimer's disease. A study of epidemiological aspects. *Ann. Neurol.*, **15**, 335–341.

Hirsch, M. J. and Wurtman, R. J. (1978). Lecithin consumption elevates acetylcholine concentrations in rat brain and adrenal gland. *Science*, **202**, 223–225.

Jarvik, L. F. and Matsuyama, S. S. (1983). Parental stroke: a risk factor for multi-infarct dementia? *Lancet*, **2**, 1025.

Kay, D. W. K., Beamish, P. and Roth, M. (1962). Some medical and social characteristics of elderly people under state care, in P. Halvos (Ed.), *The Sociological Review*. Monograph No. 5, 173–193. Keele.

Kay, D. W. K., Beamish, P. and Roth, M. (1964). Old age mental disorders in Newcastle upon Tyne. *Brit. J. Psychiat.*, **110**, 146–158.

Kay, D. W. K., Bergman, K., Foster, E. M., McKechnie, A. A. and Roth, M. (1970). Mental illness and hospital usage in the elderly: a random sample followed up. *Compr. Psychiat.*, **11**, 26–35.

Larsson, T., Sjogren, T. and Jacobson, G. (1963) Senile dementia — summary and conclusions. *Acta. Psychiat. Scand.*, **39**, suppl. 167, 215–227.

Mayer-Gross, W., Slater, E. and Roth, M. (1969). In *Clinical Psychiatry*, 3rd Edn. Baillière, Tindall and Cassell, London.

Mahendra, B. (1984). Some ethical issues in dementia research. *J. Med. Ethics*, **10**, (1), 29–31.

Melnick, V. L., Dubler, N. N., Weisbard, A. and Butler, R. N. (1984). Clinical research in senile dementia of the Alzheimer type — guidelines addressing ethical and legal issues. *J. Am. Geriat. Soc.*, **32** (7), 531–536.

Pattie, A. H. (1981). A survey version of the Clifton Assessment Procedures for the Elderly. *Brit. J. Clin. Psychol.*, **20**, 173–178.

Perry, E. K., Tomlinson, B. E., Blessed, G., Bergmann, K., Gibson, P. H., and Perry, R. H. (1978). Correlation of cholinergic abnormalities with senile plaques and mental test scores in senile dementia. *Brit. Med. J.*, **2**, 1457–1459.

Piper, M. (1979). Practical aspects of psychometric testing in the elderly. *Age Ageing*, **8**, 299–302.

Raichle, M. E., Grubb, R. L., Gado, M. H., Eichling, J. O. and Ter Pogossian, M. M. (1976). Correlation between regional cerebral blood flow and oxidative metabolism. *Arch. Neurol.*, **33**, 523–526.

Ratcliffe, P. J. and Wilcock, G. K. (1985). Cerebrovascular disease in dementia. The importance of atrial fibrillation. *Post-grad. Med. J.*, **61**, 201–204.

Roth, M. and Iversen, L. L. (Eds) (1986). Alzheimer's disease and related disorders. *Brit. Med. Bull.*, **42** (1).

Sanford, J. R. A. (1975). Tolerance of debility in elderly dependants by supporters at home: its significance for hospital practice. *Brit. Med. J.*, **3**, 471–473.

Schlesselman, J. J. (1973a). Planning a longitudinal study: 1. Sample size determination. *J. Chron. Dis.*, **26**, 553–560.

Schlesselman, J. J. (1973b). Planning a longitudinal study: 2. Frequency of measurement and study duration. *J. Chron. Dis.*, **26**, 561–570.

Small, G. W. and Jarvik, L. F. (1982). The dementia syndrome. *Lancet*, **2**, 1443–1446.

Smith, J. and Kiloh, L. G. (1981). The investigation of dementia: results in 200 consecutive admissions. *Lancet*, **1**, 824–827.

Strachan, R. W. and Henderson, J. G. (1965). Psychiatric syndromes due to avitaminosis B_{12} with normal blood and marrow. *Quart. J. Med.*, **34**, 303–317.

Sussman, M. B. (1964). Use of the longitudinal design in studies of long-term illness: some advantages and limitations. *Gerontologist*, **4**, 25–29.

Terry, R. H. (1985). Some unanswered questions about the mechanisms and aetiology of Alzheimer's disease. *Dan. Med. Bull.*, **32**, Suppl. 1, 22–24.

Thomas, D. J., Marshall, J., Ross-Russell, R. W., Wetherley-Mein, G., DuBoulay, G. H., Pearson, T. C. and Symon, L. Z. (1977). Effect of haematocrit on cerebral blood flow in man. *Lancet*, **2**, 941–943.

Wells, N. E. J. (1979). *Dementia in Old Age*. Office of Health Economics, London.

Wood, R. T. and Holden, U. P. (1982). Reality orientation, in B. Isaacs (Ed.), *Recent Advances in Geriatric Medicine, II, NY*, pp. 181–199. Churchill Livingstone.

Wright, A. F. and Whalley, L. J. (1984). The demented elderly admitted to a psychogeriatric unit. *Brit. J. Psychiat.*, **145**, 20–38.

Wroe, D. C. L. (1978). Ageing and public expenditure in the United Kingdom, in V. Carver and P. Liddiard (Eds), *An Ageing Population*. Hodder & Stoughton in association with the Open University Press.

Index